THE
SOUND
— OF —
HER VOICE

THE
SOUND

— OF —

HER VOICE

MY BLIND PARENTS' STORY

MARY PIERONI HARPER

Printed in the United States of America.
First paperback edition September 2022.

Cover and layout design by G Sharp Design, LLC.
www.gsharpmajor.com

ISBN 978-0-578-38182-4 (paperback)
Library of Congress Control Number: 2022917526

In memory of my parents, Mario and Jane Pieroni
Though their world was dark, they spread light and love

NOTE TO THE READER

MY PARENTS HAD no idea what I looked like. They'd never seen me, my sisters and brother, or even each other. Both of my parents were completely blind. Their world was totally dark, yet they independently raised four sighted children. My mother ran the household, and my father was a successful attorney and judge.

This book is based upon transcripts of interviews and tape recordings that my parents made, telling the stories of their lives. My own memories, along with my siblings' recollections, help to round out the book. The extraordinary number of newspaper and magazine articles written about my parents over eight decades also provided different perspectives, allowing me to perceive my family from an outsider's vantage.

I am often asked what it was like to grow up with blind parents. I explain in Part Two that they did the things ordinary people do, just in a different way. My parents took excellent care of me, loved me and provided for all my material needs. I didn't take care of them, although I had responsibilities that other kids didn't have, such as walking with and guiding them or checking for spots on their clothing.

Despite the constant challenges, they lived full and gracious lives. Both of my parents are gone now, but I hope that their story will inspire others and show that being blind doesn't have to mean a marginalized life.

CONTENTS

Note: Braille numbers are used at the beginning of
each chapter instead of print numbers.

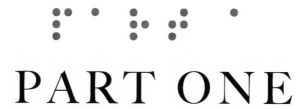

PART ONE

•

A RARE EVENT: SEPTEMBER 9, 1913

IN THE CRAMPED farmhouse bedroom, Bessie Small smiled happily as she prepared to hold her newborn daughter for the first time, but her expression quickly turned to horror when she saw the baby's grossly enlarged eyes.

"What's wrong with her eyes?" A surge of fear rose through her body. Her child's blue eyes were almost too big for their sockets. Bessie looked up at the doctor for answers. Dr. Jewett had delivered Bessie herself twenty-eight years earlier and was a trusted advisor.

"You need to rest, Bessie," he replied. "Your labor was long and difficult. Your baby is beautiful and healthy—there's nothing to worry about. Here's some medicine that will help you sleep."

"No! I don't want to sleep! There's something wrong with her eyes!" Bessie anxiously looked from the doctor to her husband, Charles. "They don't look right. Her eyeballs are too big."

"Yes," the doctor agreed. "I'm not sure what's wrong. She might have an eye disease."

"Can't you do something?" begged Bessie, her face drawn in pain and fear.

"I'm sorry, I can't. Perhaps fluid built up inside her eyes while she was in the womb, and it couldn't drain. Then her eyes swelled up and pressed on the optic nerve. But that's just a guess. I don't really know."

"Oh my God! Is she blind?"

"It's too soon to tell. This is a very rare condition. There's nothing that I can do now, but I'll write to an Indianapolis colleague to see if he has any ideas. I'm sorry. I wish that I could help more."

Bessie looked frantically in disbelief, shifting her gaze from her child's eyes to the doctor's eyes, searching for reassurance, answers—anything that would stop the nightmare. A tidal wave of nausea welled up as she fought to fully grasp what the doctor was saying. She stared at Charles, wondering how he could be so calm. Their baby might be blind! How could he just stand there?

The doctor looked at Charles. "Take care of your wife and baby. I'll let you know when I hear back from the specialist." Dr. Jewett picked up his leather bag and let himself out into the early morning darkness of the quiet Indiana countryside.

During the following weeks, both parents anxiously waited for news from Dr. Jewett while trying to maintain a normal routine. Bessie nursed her baby, named Ella Jane, giving Bessie time to study her beautiful child's swollen eyes as they looked up at her. Would the distention ever subside? Could Ella Jane even see her mother's face? Did her eyes hurt? She didn't cry excessively, and Bessie hoped that she was not in pain. She tried not to think too much about a future with a blind child.

As Bessie washed diapers by hand in a wooden washtub, she relived her pregnancy, trying to find a cause for her baby's grotesque eyes. Turning the handle to move the tub's agitator paddles, she watched the diapers swish in the water. Bessie remembered the nausea she'd suffered for months. She hadn't been so sick with her first child. Maybe that was what had caused it.

Bessie ran each clean diaper through the wringer, squeezing the water out. Gathering the laundry in a wicker basket, she recalled the fall she had taken just weeks before giving birth.

She'd missed a step outside the back door. Her friend had a stillborn baby after she had fallen. Bessie didn't think that her fall could have caused swollen eyes, but anything was possible. In the back yard at the clothesline, she sighed while hanging diapers one by one, clipping them to the line with wooden pins and praying for her baby's eyes to become normal.

Back inside the farmhouse living room, Bessie smiled as she watched her three-year-old daughter, Irma, gently rocking Ella Jane in her cradle.

"Baa, baa black sheep, have you any wool? Yes sir, yes sir, three bags full," Irma sang softly to her sister, watching her face and studying the baby's eyes. "Mother, why do her eyes look so big? Can she see me?"

"I don't know why her eyes are so big. We're waiting to hear what the doctor in Indianapolis says, but I think that she can still see you. She loves her big sister."

Bessie forced a reassuring smile and hugged her daughter, wondering how she would manage if Ella Jane was blind. Would she have to watch her every minute, so she wouldn't hurt herself? How could she get her work done if she had to worry that Ella Jane might trip and fall or bump into the table and knock over a lit kerosene lamp? At least now the baby couldn't move on her own, so Bessie had some time to figure out how to keep her safe. Then she said a silent prayer that Ella Jane's eyes would be all right.

That evening, Bessie stood at the old wood stove, stirring a pot of soup. The back door slammed, and she looked up to see Charles wearily cross the kitchen. He kissed her cheek, then sighed as he sat down to remove his shoes.

"You look awfully tired, Charles. You worry me out there in the fields by yourself all day," said Bessie.

"You know that I don't mind being alone. Besides, I have old Paint to keep me company.

That horse is a good listener."

Bessie laughed. "Does he give you advice?"

"No, no. He doesn't say much. But sometimes I like to tell him about my troubles."

Bessie's smile faded. "Your troubles? You mean that you're worried about Ella Jane?" "Well, yes, of course. I love both of my daughters, but girls can't help me much on the farm. And now if Ella Jane does go blind, how could she learn to be a housewife? She couldn't cook. And who would want to marry her?" Charles exhaled a long breath. "We'll have to support her all her life. I don't know what will happen to her when we die."

"Now, Charles. Stop thinking like that. We don't even know how bad her eyes are yet. Maybe there's something that the doctor in Indianapolis can do for her. Go wash up. Dinner is almost ready."

Two weeks later, Dr. Jewett drove his horse and buggy to the Small home. Bessie answered his knock on the door, looking expectantly for any sign of good news. The doctor smiled at Bessie, but his expression gave away nothing.

"Hello, Dr. Jewett. Please come in and have a seat. I'll find Charles. I know that he'll want to hear what you have to say."

While Bessie cradled Ella Jane in her arms, Charles sat down next to them on the couch.

Laughing, Irma climbed up onto her father's lap and touched his face. Charles smiled but removed her hand and shushed her.

The doctor cleared his throat and began the conversation that he'd been dreading.

"Bessie and Charles, I've received a letter from my colleague in Indianapolis. You know that he's studied the eye for many years and is an expert in the field. I'm sorry to say that Ella Jane's swollen eyes are most likely caused by glaucoma. There is no cure."

Bessie gasped. "You mean that she's going to be blind? There's nothing that you can do?"

"I'm so sorry. I wish that there was something that we could do. In fact, my colleague said to tell you not to sell everything you own to look for a cure. Don't waste your money going to other doctors. Some parents do that, and they end up with nothing and still have a blind child."

Bessie looked down at her baby's bloated eyes and struggled to hold back her tears. It was almost impossible to comprehend that her beautiful daughter would someday be blind.

Bessie felt her world collapsing; the unspoken fears for her daughter's future had come true. As Bessie realized that nothing could be done, she vowed to do everything possible to make Ella Jane the happiest baby in the county.

While Bessie made the vow with the best of intentions, and Ella Jane was indeed a happy baby, her happiness did not last. Her eyes grew worse in childhood. Bessie often reminded Ella Jane of her limitations, but her efforts to protect her daughter only motivated Ella

Jane to prove to her mother and others that she was capable of much more than sitting around and being waited upon.

:

THREE SISTERS

As ELLA JANE grew and learned to walk, Bessie kept a constant vigil on her daughter. She worried about her safety, though her older daughter, Irma, was usually right beside her watching to make sure that her sister didn't toddle too close to the woodstove or reach for a lit kerosene lamp. Bessie couldn't tell how much sight Ella Jane had, though it was evident that the baby had some vision. She reached for objects, and her face lit up when Charles came into the room, calling, "Dada!"

Bessie enjoyed watching Irma read Mother Goose stories to her sister. Ella Jane would happily point out objects in pictures, reassuring Bessie that although her daughter's eyes bulged, she could still see.

Bessie and Charles welcomed their third daughter, Ruth, when Ella Jane was almost three years old. Just days after Ruth's birth, Ella Jane begged her mother for permission to hold her baby sister. Bessie feared Ella Jane might drop the baby, but Ella Jane insisted that she would be careful. Bessie couldn't hold back a smile when Ella Jane sat on the couch, gently holding the baby while making silly faces and sounds to quiet her fussy sister.

While Bessie ironed the family's laundry or cleaned the house, she enjoyed stopping occasionally to watch her two older daughters play school. Irma, at age seven, was the teacher since Ella Jane was too young to go to school. Despite not being able to see clearly, Ella Jane tried hard to imitate her sister's printing of the alphabet. She told Bessie that she could hardly wait until she would be old enough to join Irma at the school in Lincolnville; she desperately wanted to be like her big sister and read her own books. When Irma left for school, Bessie saw how bored and lonely Ella Jane was without her sister's company. Ella Jane played with Ruth while waiting for Irma to return, but Bessie could tell by Ella Jane's face how happy she was to hear Irma walking up the gravel driveway.

Ella Jane was fiercely independent from a very young age. She wanted to tie her own shoes, not have her mother tie them for her. She insisted on picking out which dress to wear each day. Details of a fabric design, such as small flowers, were hard for her to see, but she could see the color and knew each dress by feeling the material.

When she was only five years old, her aunt, Mary Ella, caught her eating a cookie before dinner and loudly chastised her. Ella Jane told Bessie she didn't want to share her name with her mean aunt, that "Ella is my aunt's name, not mine. My name is Jane." After that declaration, Bessie and the rest of her family were careful to only call her Jane. Even as an adult, if an official government document arrived addressed to Ella Jane, she'd sniff and say with an offended tone, "Ella is not my name. Why do they have to use that awful name?"

As the girls got older, Bessie decided that Irma and Jane could gather eggs from the hen house. She had shown them how to get the eggs out of the nest without getting nipped by an angry hen, but the girls were still apprehensive the first time they tried it without their mother.

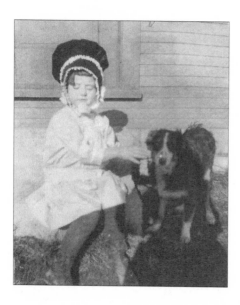

Jane and her dog, Billy

"Irma, you go first. Grab her by the tail and throw her off. Then I'll get the eggs," said Jane.

Irma knocked the squawking hen off her nest while Jane reached up, feeling for the eggs. The indignant chicken rose, noisily flapping its wings at Jane's face and body. She waved her free hand, batting at the angry bird.

"Ow! Stupid old chicken! Get away from me! Here, Irma, take these eggs and put them in the basket," said Jane as she carefully plucked the eggs from the nest and handed them to her sister. "Then hurry up and get the next one off her nest. I hate getting these eggs. These chickens are mean."

Irma stamped her feet and waved her arms in a vain attempt to push the aggressive birds away from her sister. By the time she'd pulled each chicken off its nest, the hen house was awash in flying feathers, flapping wings, and screeching, protesting chickens.

"Let's go! I don't care if I didn't get all the eggs. Mom can get them. Ouch! That chicken just scratched my arm," said Jane. She couldn't get out of the hen house fast enough.

Irma loved being Jane's sister. The two were inseparable during the summer and played with their dolls or held tea parties under the tall elm tree. They loved to play tag in the yard. Jane could see well enough to find good hiding places, and Irma delighted in finding her. But when Irma was seven, she began to feel pain in her knees whenever she ran. The pain didn't stop her from running, but sometimes Irma had to slow down and rest.

For as long as Irma remembered she had called her father "Pop," as did her other sisters.

When he didn't need Old Paint, the family's horse, he allowed Irma and Jane to go for bareback rides. Of course, Irma would be in charge, yet she knew that Jane wanted to be just like her and ride in the front so that she could steer the horse.

One sunny June day, Pop put the bridle on the horse, then helped Irma climb up, followed by Jane.

"Be careful, girls. Don't go too far! And don't let Jane steer the horse," Pop warned. "She might steer him into something and have an accident."

"Yes, Pop. We'll be careful," Irma promised.

Charles gently tapped Old Paint's rump, and he began a slow ramble out of the barnyard. The girls settled in for a leisurely ride, with Jane's arms circling Irma's middle. After riding a few minutes down the quiet country road, Irma turned and looked for her father.

"Jane, I don't see him! Do you want to steer?" Irma knew that they were disobeying their father, but Irma was confident that Jane could handle the responsibility.

"Oh yes! You know I'd love to steer Old Paint. Can we switch places?"

"Okay," said Irma as she brought the horse to a stop. "You hold onto my shoulders and stand up. Now swing your leg over my shoulder!"

After much twisting and turning, while Irma tried not to cry out from her knee pain, Jane finally got settled in front of her sister and took the reins. She turned her head around and grinned at her sister. For Irma, Jane's smile was the best. Jane turned back, shook the reins, and said, "Let's go, Old Paint!"

The horse ambled on down the dirt road. A half-mile later, they passed their neighbor's house and waved to their friends, two sisters who often came over to play. Irma knew that Jane was enjoying her ride but realized that she could no longer tolerate the pain throbbing in her knees.

"Jane, my knees are hurting again. This old horse makes them bounce and I don't want to ride anymore."

"But we haven't been riding for very long!" Jane protested. "All right. We'll go back. Shall we trade places again? I don't want Pop to see me steering Old Paint." They repeated their earlier twisting and turning as Jane moved behind Irma, who couldn't keep back the tears as pain shot through both knees.

In the days that followed, the swelling and redness in Irma's knees did not subside. Walking became painful. The same doctor who had delivered Irma, Dr. Jewett, diagnosed her with rheumatism and said that he was sorry, but the only things he could suggest were rest and a hot water bottle on her joints. Irma tried to be brave as her mother rubbed liniment onto her knees, using the same bottle that Pop used to help Old Paint when he was lame. Despite the label's promise of relief, it did nothing to stop Irma's pain.

It became more difficult for Irma to keep up with her younger sisters as they climbed tall trees and roamed the woods. She watched as they laughed and had adventures without her, and she felt left out and alone.

Life on the farm revolved around the seasons, with spring bringing planting time and canning season in the late summer. Although there was plenty of work to be done, Jane's parents would not let the girls help. They decided that Irma, now ten years old, and Ruth, age four, should watch seven-year-old Jane, instead of being required to do many chores. When Irma couldn't join them outside, Ruth was trusted by their parents to keep Jane safe.

Early on a summer morning, the girls were awakened by the sounds of horses and wagons arriving in the backyard and men's voices shouting instructions as they unloaded wood from their wagons. This was a special day on the Small farm, one that the sisters had eagerly anticipated.

The men were there to help build Pop's new barn. Every day Jane and her sisters watched with excitement as the men built the structure, install outside posts, and form the peak of the roof. Narrow beams connected the posts to hold the structure steady. Already the girls were planning where to play in the new structure and hoped that Pop would let them make a little house up in the hayloft.

Late one afternoon, after the workers had gone home, Jane and Ruth found a ladder that had been left propped against the base of the barn's skeleton.

"Jane, look! There's a ladder! Let's climb it." Jane knew that Ruth loved to climb trees, furniture, or anything that allowed her to be off the ground, so she wasn't surprised that Ruth wanted to climb it.

Seven-year-old Jane and four-year-old Ruth ran to the barn. Without hesitation, Jane followed Ruth up the ladder. At the top, Ruth stepped out onto the narrow beam, high above the ground. But Jane stopped. She couldn't see where to step. Maybe this wasn't such a good idea after all.

Ruth held out her hand. "Here, Jane, put your hand on the wood. See, that's where you put your feet." Ruth took her hand and put it down on the beam. Jane moved her hand from one side of the beam to the other. It felt awfully narrow, but Ruth seemed to fit okay, so she climbed off the ladder and onto the beam, her arms wobbling as she sought her balance. Together they slowly inched along and eventually arrived at the end, where they held on to a post that would hold up the roof.

"What do you see, Ruth?"

"We're up real high," said Ruth. "I see the pigs."

"I can smell 'em. I don't have to see the pigs. I know that they're just below us."

"I see chickens, too. They look so tiny." Even at Ruth's young age, Jane depended on her little sister to describe the world to her.

"I can hear them clucking, but I can't really see them. Maybe we ought to go back now." Jane had begun to feel a little frightened as she realized how high up she was. She tightened her grip on her sister's small hand. Balancing on the beam, they slowly made their way back to the ladder. Jane carefully used her right foot to find each rung of the ladder, making her way toward the ground.

When both feet touched the soft earth, she finally relaxed and heaved a sigh of relief.

Running to the barn, Bessie and Charles met the girls at the bottom of the ladder. They had been watching, horror-stricken and helpless, from the kitchen window. They knew that if they had yelled at their daughters, they could have fallen to their deaths. Jane saw her mother shaking with fear before she pulled Ruth and her into a hug. Jane promised that they would never climb up there again. She expected to be punished, but her parents were so relieved that they were safe, they forgot to discipline the girls.

After that day, Charles vigilantly secured all ladders and locked the barnyard gate. The girls could have climbed over the gate and fences, but after realizing how much they had scared their parents, didn't want to push their luck.

Since Irma's rheumatism prevented her from riding Old Paint, Pop made Jane wait until Ruth was old enough to go riding with her. One hot afternoon in August, when Ruth was five and Jane was eight, the girls decided to go for a ride.

"Pop? Can Jane and I go for a ride on Old Paint?" asked Ruth. Both sisters knew that Irma wouldn't be able to ride. Jane watched as Ruth glanced at Irma with a look of feigned pity. Jane knew that Ruth liked being able to do something that Irma couldn't do. Irma was older and read a lot of books, but Ruth had more fun doing active things around the farm.

"Alright, come on. I'll get the bridle on for you," Pop said as he headed out the back door.

Jane was the first to climb up on the horse's back. Pop had long ago watched as Jane guided the horse and realized that even with her very limited vision, it was safe for her to steer. Old Paint knew the area well, and he could be counted on to come back, even without being told.

Pop helped Ruth up and made sure that she was comfortable behind her sister.

"Bye, Pop! Let's go, Old Paint!" Jane urged the horse on. The gentle horse sauntered out of the barnyard, but Jane didn't mind the pace. She didn't want the horse to trot or gallop, as that would have been too scary given her poor vision.

As the girls passed by the front porch, Ruth waved and yelled, "Hi Irma! This is fun!" Irma looked up from her book and waved back, though she didn't smile at her younger sisters. Jane knew it was hard for her to sit in pain while they were out enjoying a ride. She felt somewhat guilty leaving her behind and wished that her beloved sister didn't have to suffer, but she was glad that Ruth was finally old enough to ride with her.

After a pleasant ride through the fields, it was time to return home. Ruth became impatient. "Jane let's take a shortcut through the orchard. I'm hungry, and I want to go home."

"Alright. I think that I see it just up ahead," Jane said as she guided the horse toward the blurry trees. At age eight, her sight had continued to slowly fade, but Jane didn't let her worsening vision stop her from enjoying her rides on Old Paint.

Moments later, she heard a crunch and felt apple tree branches scraping her arms and leaves tapping her face. Her hands dropped the reins as she tried to push away the foliage, getting more scratched while she struggled to back away.

"Ouch! Bad horse!" She found the reins and pulled back, trying to disentangle from the madding branches. "Ruth, why didn't you tell me that I was going to run into a tree?"

"I can't see around you. Besides, I thought that you could see that big ol' tree!"

Jane was embarrassed that she hadn't seen the tree. She never had a problem going through the orchard before that day. Jane realized that she was going to have to be more careful. Feeling her arms, she was relieved to find two thin, angry scratches but no sticky blood.

"Don't tell Pop that I didn't see the tree. He'll get upset and might not let us ride anymore." Jane feared losing more than just the horse rides. Pop worried about everything that she did.

Roller skating on the front porch. Running through the fields. Playing down by the creek. He wouldn't let the girls have bicycles, claiming that they only had two wheels for balancing, whereas horses had four feet and were safer than bicycles. He didn't allow Irma and Ruth to have bicycles because he knew that Jane would ride them. If she ever hurt herself, she worried that he would make her stay home with Irma. While she loved playing with her older sister, Jane didn't want to just sit around.

"As soon as we get home, I'm going to put on a long-sleeved blouse," Jane said as she urged the horse forward. "Come on, Old Paint, let's get home."

They agreed never to tell Pop. True to her word, Ruth said nothing about the incident to their parents.

Later that summer, Jane, Irma, and Ruth sat outside on an old blanket carefully positioned under the old elm tree and arranged their dolls for their Sunday afternoon tea party.

"Jane, would you like some tea?" inquired Ruth in her best formal tone of voice.

"Why yes, please. That sounds delightful," Jane replied equally formally, then collapsed into giggles. She didn't hear her father's footsteps as he crossed the lawn and was surprised to hear him call her name.

"Jane! Please come with me."

Jane looked at her sisters and wondered if she was in trouble. Pop usually didn't interrupt their play, and she couldn't think of any reason for him to be angry with her. She got up obediently, reluctantly leaving the fun.

Pop took her hand gently and said, "Jane, I want to go for a ride in the car with you. I'm even going to let you drive it!"

Stunned, Jane looked up at her father, wondering if he was joking. She couldn't make out a smile on his face and became more confused. Why would he want her to drive?

"But, Pop! I'm only eight years old. I don't know how to drive."

"I know. You'll be sitting on my lap. You steer, and I'll give it some gas and change the gears. We'll go slowly. You'll be all right."

Still not understanding why Pop would want her to drive his expensive car, Jane hesitatingly climbed up into the passenger seat of the Ford Model T and patiently waited for him to crank up the engine. He stood in front of the car, bending over and carefully putting his hand into position on the crank. Mindful that it could buck and break a finger or his arm, he pulled the crank up and around, smiling when the engine rumbled to life.

Her father clambered up and sat behind the steering wheel, motioning Jane to join him. Once she was settled, he said, "All right. Now I want you to hold on to the steering wheel. You just keep the car on the road. Don't let it go off to the side."

The car jerked forward, startling Jane, who gripped the shaking steering wheel even harder. She felt the jiggling motion of the wheel in her hands and fought to keep the automobile on the dirt road. As they bounced along, Jane concentrated on keeping off the green grass along the road's edge. She was squinting hard just to see the grass, and between the shaking steering wheel and bouncing over rocks and ruts, Jane was exhausted after just a few minutes.

"Pop, can we stop now? I'm tired. I can't make it go straight."

"Alright," he said as he braked the car to a stop. "I'll drive us back home."

"Pop, why did you want me to drive?"

"Well, Jane, I didn't know any other way to test your vision. I figured that if you could see well enough to keep the car on the road, you still had some vision. It's just hard for me to know how much sight you still have. We'll take another drive in a few months and see if you do any worse."

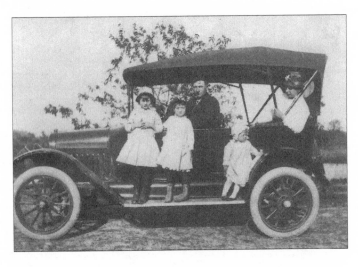

Irma, Jane, Charles, Ruth, Bessie

••

IGNORED

JANE SAT ON her bedroom floor and carefully laced up her new shoes. She felt very special wearing the pink cotton dress that her mother had made for her. Jane usually wore Irma's hand-me-downs; this dress fit just right, it wasn't too big, and the long sleeves didn't cover her hands. At age six, she felt like she'd waited her whole life for this day, and she wanted to look perfect.

Today was her first day of school, when she'd finally walk with Irma and their four neighborhood friends a half-mile down the dirt road to wait for the school "kid-hack." The open air, horse-drawn wagon would take them the three miles to school in the small crossroads community of Lincolnville, where she would meet her new teacher.

Irma winced with pain as she slowly lifted her right foot onto the high step at the back of the old wagon, then grabbed the sides and worked to pull herself up. Jane followed and sat next to her sister on the hard, wooden bench. The driver flicked the reins, and the horse started off, the wagon swaying as it lurched through dried ruts. Irma moaned quietly as each bump radiated into her body, increasing the pain. Jane heard her sister and took her hand, wishing that she could do something more to comfort her sister.

Jane was too excited to mind the rough ride. Her heart beat faster as the hack bounced its way toward the school. Jane wondered what school would be like and hoped that she would get a nice teacher. She wanted to learn to read and write. Even arithmetic problems that Irma always complained about sounded like fun. Jane smiled in anticipation.

Irma had told Jane that the school was three stories tall. It would be the biggest building that Jane had ever been in, and she was already wondering how she would find her way. When Jane entered the school still holding Irma's hand, she was quickly overwhelmed. There were students of all ages thronging the halls, with boys yelling and girls laughing as they greeted each other. Jane was not used to being around boys. The neighbor families only had girls; Jane had rarely interacted with boys her own age. Two older boys brushed past her, almost knocking her off balance. Already overcome by the noise and smells of the school, Jane clung even harder to Irma's hand as they made their way to the first-grade classroom.

Jane's new teacher, Miss Brown, greeted her at the door.

"You must be Jane Small," she said with little enthusiasm. "The principal told me that you'd be in my class this year." She stared at Jane's face. "What's wrong with your eyes? Can you see anything?"

Startled, Jane's face turned red, and she looked down at the floor, ashamed to be singled out, as if she'd already done something wrong.

"I have glaucoma," she whispered.

"What? Speak up, child! Look at me, not the floor."

"I'm sorry, Miss Brown. I can see a little. I have glaucoma."

"Well, I've never taught a child that can't see. Go on in and find your seat. Can you read your name?"

"Yes," Jane replied.

"Look for your name on your desk and sit down."

Irma whispered to Jane, "Want some help? I can go in with you." Jane nodded. "Please."

Inside the classroom, excited children chattered, but the noise stopped abruptly when Jane, lightly holding Irma's left arm, walked into the room. Feeling her classmates' eyes staring at her, Jane's pulse raced as she desperately looked for her seat.

"Here it is," said Irma, stopping at a desk at the back of the room.

Jane removed her hand from her sister's elbow and reached for the seat, feeling the smooth wood as she slid into place behind the desk.

"See you after school," Irma said as she turned to leave.

Relieved, Jane sank into the bench seat and looked around. She saw a long line of alphabet letters above the chalkboard, but she couldn't see the individual letters. Each was too blurry. She glanced at the girls sitting around her. Some smiled, while others continued to stare at her eyes.

Miss Brown closed the door and walked to the front of the classroom. The unusually tall teacher wore a black dress that accented her thin figure and crisply told the children to sit up straight and stop talking. Jane's formal education had begun.

It was hard for Jane to distinguish her teacher's facial expressions; she relied upon auditory clues to determine Miss Brown's mood. The teacher sighed frequently, as if teaching the class of farm children was an impossible task. She rarely smiled and gave little encouragement to the students. Rules were strict, and mischievous students were put in the corner facing the wall. Jane was frightened of her teacher and kept very quiet, not daring to break a rule.

Jane struggled to see what Miss Brown wrote on the distant chalkboard. Whether the teacher wrote letters or numbers, it was all a blur to

Jane. If she squeezed her eyes, she could see the shape a little better. But that was very tiring. Jane quickly grew frustrated with her inability to see the chalkboard. Nobody else seemed to have difficulty seeing what the teacher wrote. She hated feeling different from the other children and wished that she could ask Miss Brown to move her up to the first row, but she was too frightened to approach the stern woman.

When Miss Brown passed out primers with simple words in large print, Jane hoped that she would be able to see the letters. She was elated when she realized that the print was large enough for her see, although it was still fuzzy. Jane couldn't see well up close or far away, and despite her desire to learn and persistence, she fell behind her classmates.

One day Jane finally mustered up the courage to raise her hand. "Miss Brown, I need some help, please. I can't see what you are writing on the board," said Jane.

"I have to help all the other children. You can't see, so I don't know how you'll ever learn to read. Here's a book with pictures. Surely you can look at those pictures. Keep quiet, now. You're taking time away from everyone who can see."

Humiliated, Jane felt her cheeks redden and a lump rise in her throat. She struggled not to cry as she wondered, *Why doesn't the teacher like me? Why won't she help me? Everyone else is learning to print. I know that I can use a pencil, but I can't see the letters that she writes on the board. I can't copy them if I can't see them. Every day I get farther and farther behind. I'll never read or write. Maybe I'm just too stupid to learn.*

Jane strained her eyes trying to do the work. Every day she arrived home with pounding headaches, and wouldn't tell her mother. She thought it was her own fault that she couldn't see. She was bored and frustrated at school, but it was still better than staying home all day. Her mother wouldn't let her do much at home because she was afraid that she might get hurt. School was her chance to do something—anything—but first grade was a big disappointment.

Her only solace was recess when she was released from the uncomfortable wooden seat and desk. Jane and her two best friends, Helen and Dorothy, relished their time on the playground. Helen often pushed Jane on a swing, with Jane stretching her legs up into the air as far as she could, laughing as she pretended to be flying.

One day, tiring of the swing, Jane jumped off and said, "Let's play a game of tag! Dorothy, you're it!"

The girls squealed and darted in different directions. Jane had no trouble running and easily kept her balance on the uneven grass. She'd played tag many times with her sisters and had no fear of running into something. The freedom she felt while forgetting her classroom limitations helped to make the day bearable.

Suddenly, two third-grade boys stepped in front of Jane as she was trying to escape Dorothy's tag. She stumbled into their outstretched arms and cried out, "Oh! What are you doing? Get out of my way!"

"I thought that you were blind. How can you run?" asked the bigger boy.

"Yeah, you can't run if you can't see. You must not be blind," echoed the second child.

"Let me go! Leave me alone!" Jane twisted her body, flailing her arms as she worked free of the boys' grip.

"Well, you sure have ugly eyes!" Both boys laughed loudly, turned, and ran off, leaving Jane shaking where she stood.

Dorothy had stopped a few feet away, watching in horror as her friend struggled with the boys. After they were gone, she approached

Jane and put her arm around her shoulders. "Those boys are stupid and horrible! I'm sorry that they were so mean to you. At least they're not in our class."

Although first grade was a wasted year for Jane, second grade was much better. Her new teacher, Miss Starr, liked Jane and wanted to help. Although she did not have specific training for teaching a blind child, she was a creative teacher who thought of practical techniques to help.

Jane was given a front row desk, allowing for frequent interaction with her teacher. Miss Starr wrote in large letters on the chalkboard and invited Jane to move closer as needed. With Miss Starr's kindness and patience, Jane flourished and caught up with her classmates.

By the third grade, though, Jane's vision worsened, and the print looked even dimmer.

She couldn't see to read, and although she tried hard, she once again fell behind. Every afternoon her head pounded with the strain of sitting for hours trying to discern letters. Desperately wanting to learn and frustrated that her eyes weren't functioning, each day, she felt increasingly despondent. Unlike the compassionate Miss Starr, her third-grade teacher was not sympathetic and made no effort to adjust her teaching methods.

At home one afternoon, Charles said to Jane, "I've noticed how sad you are when you come home from school."

A tear trickled down Jane's cheek. "Pop, I just can't see. And my teacher won't help me because she says that she's too busy."

"I think that I should go down and talk to the superintendent. Maybe he'll know what to do. Would you like that?"

Jane nodded her head. Pop's words gave her hope. But when he came home from the meeting, that hope faded much like her eyesight.

The superintendent had told Pop that he was sympathetic as he, too, had a handicap; he'd returned from World War I with an amputated arm. He recognized Jane's problem and suggested to Pop that perhaps someone could read to Jane, but he knew that wouldn't solve all her problems. He was sorry, but his teachers were doing all that they could for Jane.

On a warm spring afternoon, Jane and Irma climbed down from the school wagon, said goodbye to their friends, and walked slowly toward home. Jane's head pounded from a long day of straining to see. The bright sun in the cloudless sky added to her pain, but she didn't want to complain to Irma. Irma's knees were hurting—she could tell by the sound of her sister's limp as they walked down the dirt road. Yet Jane felt like crying as she remembered her teacher's harsh words earlier that afternoon. It wasn't her fault that she couldn't keep up with the class. Why couldn't anyone help her?

As Bessie cleared the dinner dishes from the table that evening, Jane stayed at the table. "I asked my teacher for help today with reading," Jane said. "But she told me, 'Well, you can't see, so you can't do what everyone else is doing. That's just the way it is.'" A tear escaped from her eyes and Jane continued, "It makes me feel so bad. I'm trying, but I just can't see the print. And my head hurts all the time. I loved school in second grade, but now I hate it."

Through her blurred vision she saw Pop look at her mother, who nodded as she poured a bucket of water into the sink. "Jane," he said, "I was at the bank a couple of weeks ago. The teller asked about you. I told her that you weren't happy, and she told me that she'd heard about a school just for blind children."

"Really? A whole school for kids like me? Please let me go! I'm not learning anything now!" Jane jumped up to hug her father. "And

I wouldn't get teased or have tricks played on me anymore. Pop, when can I go?"

"After summer vacation. You will finish this year at Lincolnville. The school is in Indianapolis, so you'd have to live there. You could come home for holidays like Thanksgiving and Christmas, but most of the time you'd be at school, even on weekends."

"Oh. That means I couldn't come home every day. Where would I live?"

"They have rooms that you'd share with some other girls," answered her mother.

"That might be fun. I can make new friends. I mean, I'd miss you and Pop and Irma and Ruth. But I'd be learning and not bored like I am now."

"Pop and I will miss you. And so will Irma and Ruth. But we'll write you lots of letters," said Bessie.

But what if I get sick?"

"They will take good care of you. And if you get really sick, we'll bring you home," said Pop.

Jane had no idea where Indianapolis was or what it really meant to live away from home in a school completely different from what she'd known. She'd never been to the big city. She just knew that there was nothing for her on the farm or at school. Even her mother often told her, "You'd better let somebody else do it, because they can see." She hated being the odd one out, always having to defend herself. She just wanted to be like everyone else. At age nine, Jane knew that to have a chance of living a better life, she would have to leave her family and start over at a new school in a strange city. As scary as that was, the School for the Blind had to be better than public school in

Lincolnville. Jane's heart felt lighter, and her headache began to ease. "Mom? When can I start packing?"

..
:
.

SEPTEMBER 1924

JANE PAUSED TO look up at the large brick building, squinting as she tried to count the number of stories. "Mother, I think that I can see five stories. This is so much bigger than my school in Lincolnville!" As they climbed the steps of the Indiana School for the Blind, Jane clutched her mother's hand even tighter and wondered why she had said that she wanted to go there. She'd never been in a city, and already the sounds and smells in her new environment threatened to overwhelm her.

Arriving in the quiet admissions office, Jane fought back tears as her parents greeted the receptionist and began the paperwork that would allow them to leave her at the school. She stood silently next to Pop while he answered questions about her physical and mental condition, how much sight she had, and her previous schooling. Very few children were completely blind at the school, though all had enough impairment to prevent them from attending regular schools.

A polite but businesslike older woman took them on a brief tour of the school, which ended at Jane's new room in the girl's dormitory. Ten-year-old Jane would share her room with four other girls. She was hoping to meet her new roommates, but the room was empty. The guide showed her where her bed was located, and Pop laid her suitcase on top of it. Jane would get settled later that afternoon, but first she had to say goodbye to her parents.

As her parents hugged her, Jane felt a large lump rise slowly up her throat. She tried to swallow and force it back down. Tears formed and overflowed down her cheeks. This was it. They were going home, leaving her to stay in this enormous place with total strangers. She didn't want her parents to know how sad she was; she was afraid that they might want to take her back home. Jane watched as her parents disappeared down the hall, her mother turning once for a final wave goodbye.

Sniffling and wiping away her tears, Jane walked back to her bed and sat down. She was alone. She wouldn't see her parents again for over two months. How would she ever make it that long? Jane had never spent more than one night away from home. Now she was stuck in this strange place, missing her sisters and parents. She was tired from the trip. And getting hungry.

She didn't know what time dinner was served, or how to find the dining room. Feeling sorrier for herself by the moment, she sobbed uncontrollably.

Passing by Jane's room, another third-grade student, Marie, heard her cries. She recognized the sound of homesick tears and decided to meet the new girl.

Knocking on the door, she asked, "Hello? Can I come in?"

Turning her head to look at the fuzzy shape of a girl in a red dress, Jane wiped her tears with a handkerchief and replied, "Who are you?"

"I'm Marie. Aren't you the new girl?" Marie said as she moved toward the sound of Jane's voice.

"Yes, my parents just left. My name is Jane. You can sit next to me if you want. We don't seem to have any chairs in here." Jane patted the bed beside her, pleased to have company to distract her.

"I know. We only have beds and a chest for our clothes. Are you homesick? I got here a couple of days ago, and I'm still homesick. Can you see anything? I can see a little, but I can't read print. Maybe we can be friends," replied Marie.

"I'd like that. You're the first one that I've met. Do you like it here?"

"It's all right. The teachers are pretty nice. But the governesses can be mean unless you follow all the rules."

"What's a governess?"

"She makes sure that you brush your teeth and go to bed on time. She's sort of like a mother, except that she doesn't love you. Mostly, she tells you what to do."

"She doesn't sound very nice."

"Just do what she says and don't talk after lights out and you'll be fine. Don't expect to get any hugs from them, even if you're crying because you're homesick. They only care about you making your bed and not causing them any trouble. Say, I think that it's almost time for dinner. Want to go with me to the dining room?"

Marie took Jane's hand, and together they walked down the stairs to the dining room. On the way, Marie explained that the girls had their own dining room; boys had their own down the hall.

"You don't have to worry about being around any nasty boys. They don't eat with us.

They're only in our classes, but they sit on one side, and we sit on the other. And we can't talk to each other. We don't even play outside together," explained Marie.

"I'm glad to hear that," Jane said with relief.

Just as they entered the dining room, Jane heard a girl cry out, "There's the new girl!" and found herself surrounded by several girls who rushed over, enveloping her in a sea of hands that touched her hair, face, arms, and dress.

"What are you doing? Get your hands off me!" Jane cried as she backed away, flailing her arms in a futile effort to stop the violating hands. She instantly flashed back to the henhouse at home, when the chickens fluttered at her and flapped their wings in her face. This was even worse since she was caught off guard.

The questions flew. "What does she look like? How tall is she? Look at this dress! It's so soft. What color is it? Oh! She has short hair! And a bow in it!"

"We're just trying to see what you look like," said Dorothy. "Some of us can see a little, but others can't see at all. That's the only way we can know what you look like."

"You don't have to know what I look like. Don't touch me again," said Jane as she broke away from these new tormentors.

Marie grabbed Jane's hand and said, "Let's go sit down. I'm sorry that they did that to you. That happened to me, too. They do it to all the new girls."

Feeling violated and fearful that other girls would attack her again, Jane hesitated before sitting down with her new friend.

"Jane, sit with me. They won't bother you now. They're too busy eating. And don't worry, I won't touch you. But it would be nice to know what you look like!"

She already liked Marie and decided that it was safe to describe herself. "I'll tell you what I look like," replied Jane. "I have blue eyes and short, wavy hair that's hard to comb. I'm wearing a blue and white checked dress. I can still see some print and write a little, but not good enough for public school. That's why I'm here. There was nothing for me at my old school. Now I want to hear about you."

The girls spent the rest of the meal happily talking about their families and previous schools. They were served at their table by disinterested female employees, and Jane found the food to be very plain and bland—not at all the farm-fresh food that she was used to at home. She tried not to think about her mother's cooking—every meal reminded her of what she was missing at home, making the time until Thanksgiving vacation seem interminable.

After lunch, Jane sat on her narrow bed, feeling homesick and lost again. She dabbed a plain white handkerchief at her eyes, trying to wipe away the tears that appeared whenever she thought of her family. She even missed her old school in Lincolnville. At least she knew where everything was and didn't get lost there. She worried about finding her new classroom, if her new teacher would be nice like Miss Star, and most concerning of all, what the governesses would be like.

Marie said that though the governesses carried a paddle, they rarely used it. Instead, they often yelled at them and then reported the errant child to the superintendent. Jane shuddered at the possibility of being humiliated by the governess, who would report her to the superintendent and who, in turn, would tell her parents. She vowed to be perfectly behaved and to follow all the rules. Even though she missed her family terribly, she didn't want to go home. This was her only chance to get an education. She had to stay at school. There was nothing for her to do at home; there was no future for her on the farm.

There was a sharp knock on the door, and without waiting for an answer, a tall woman swept into Jane's room. Startled, Jane looked up and through her failing eyes saw the silhouette of a thin woman in a plain, dark gray dress, her hair pulled back into a bun.

"You must be the new girl. I'm Miss Black, and I'll be your governess. There are some things that you should know about the school and what I'm responsible for. You need to take care of your personal cleanliness. That means you take a bath by yourself every Saturday and make sure that your brush your teeth every morning and night. You will dress yourself. I don't have time to put dresses on every girl."

Opening a drawer in Jane's dresser, she said, "Make your bed neatly every morning. And put away your clothes. Don't leave anything on the floor. We don't want anyone tripping over shoes or a piece of clothing that you're too lazy to pick up."

Jane watched the woman and wondered why she was looking in her drawer.

"I see that you have folded your blouses very neatly. I think that you must be a very tidy girl. Always be tidy. It will help you to find things because they will always be where they should be. None of this throwing clothing into a drawer and slamming it shut business."

"When you're walking in the hall or going down the stairs, always stay to the right," she continued. "That way, you won't run into another student. You will find the dining room, classroom, and playrooms by yourself. Can you see at all?"

Overwhelmed, Jane nodded weakly.

Miss Black crossed the room and stood by the door. "Well, I don't know how much you can see, but if you get lost, you can ask another girl. Just don't ask a boy. Boys and girls are not allowed to talk to each other. Any questions?" She turned to leave, her hand on the doorknob.

"No, Miss Black."

"Well, I'll be watching you. If you follow the rules, you'll be just fine." The door shut behind her, leaving Jane alone once again.

Stunned, Jane fought back tears. Another wave of homesickness struck her as she thought about her mother and her loving hugs. Miss

Black wasn't going to comfort her. Marie was a friend who commiserated with her, but it was clear that she'd have to make it on her own. She had no other choice.

It took Jane just a couple of days to become familiar with the layout of the school. She listened for the sound of shoes tapping down steps and knew that the stairs were close by.

Walking down the halls, she ran her right hand along the rough plaster walls. When her hand hit air, that indicated an open door. If her hand felt wood, the door was closed. She counted the number of doors until she knew how many she needed to pass before reaching her destination. To find the bathroom, she turned right from her room and counted two doors. The third door was their communal bath.

Jane adapted easily to indoor plumbing and never missed the outhouse at home. Baths were allowed on Saturdays; Jane enjoyed the warm water and the heated bathrooms. She was used to bathing in a tin tub in the chilly kitchen of her farmhouse. With no running water, Bessie would pump buckets full of cold water at the well and heat it on the wood stove. By the time it was Jane's turn to get into the tub, the water was chilly and dirty. Here, the baths at school were luxurious with warm water right out of the faucet.

Only a few students were completely blind. Most had low vision and could read fairly well, although they were not able to see well enough to attend public schools. Jane could still read and write letters when she first arrived at Indianapolis. Telephones were not common in the mid-1920s, so the only way for people to communicate was by letter. Getting a letter from home was always an exciting event. When the mail arrived, those with some vision read the letters out loud to the recipients. Of course, there was no privacy in that system. Children who didn't get letters hung around and listened to another family's news. It was better than nothing for those unlucky ones.

At the beginning of the school year, Jane was placed in the third grade. Her favorite part of the day was when the teacher, Miss Jenkins, read books such as *The Adventures of Huckleberry Finn* and *Raggedy Ann* to the class, which helped to inspire a lifelong love of literature.

While listening to stories engaged her imagination, Jane's world expanded greatly when she learned Braille. Sitting at a small table equipped with a pegboard, she made Braille letters and numbers by putting pegs into the holes. Each letter and number have a distinctive pattern, and she practiced all thirty-six patterns. Once she could easily and quickly make every letter, she made simple words on the pegboard.

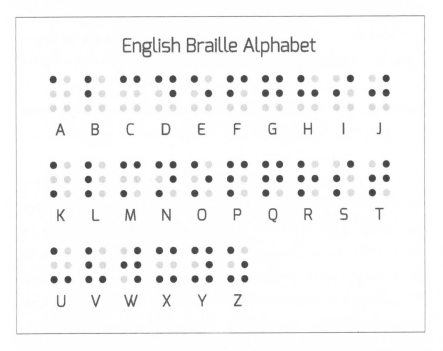

"Jane, I think that you're ready to start reading a Braille book," said Miss Jenkins as she put a copy of *Mother Goose Rhymes* in her hands.

"You've already started making and reading words on the pegboard. This will be easier than the pegboard. Please open the book and start reading to me on the first page."

Jane tentatively put her fingers on the dots, feeling each one while moving her fingers to follow the dots across the page.

"J-a-c-k," Jane spelled aloud. "Jack!" Jane's face lit up with the realization that her world was about to grow much larger and exciting. Soon she'd be able to read by herself and not have to depend upon others to read to her.

"That's right, Jane. Very good. As you practice, you'll go faster, and you'll recognize words like 'and' and 'the' without thinking so hard. You'll be reading chapter books before you know it," encouraged Miss Jenkins.

Jane reveled in the teacher's attention; she had been ignored so often in public school that she'd almost given up learning anything. She blossomed under the kind, patient instructor. No longer was she frustrated and humiliated in the classroom, unable to keep up with the sighted students in Lincolnville. School became fun for Jane, and she eagerly looked forward to class.

While she worked at mastering reading, Jane learned how to write Braille using a slate and stylus. She opened the slate and inserted the special, thick paper—thin paper made for sloppy and illegible dots—and squeezed the two ends of the slate together. Now the paper was gripped tightly and wouldn't slip when she punched holes. Next, she held the stylus with the sharp end down and used the small cells within the slate to guide her hand as she punched the dots into the paper that became letters. Jane quickly learned how to read and write Braille, a skill that she would use in school for taking notes and answering test questions. It also enabled her to enjoy a lifetime of reading and made daily life easier by using Braille labels for clothes and canned foods.

After class one day, Jane and her friends walked down to the mailroom, hoping that a letter from home would be waiting.

"Jane, here's a letter for you," said the woman behind the desk.

"Thank you," she replied, holding out her hand. With the precious paper held tightly, Jane moved to the back and waited for her friends to learn if they'd get an envelope.

When the letters had been distributed, Jane asked, "Can somebody read this to me?"

"I can. I didn't get anything today," Molly said sadly.

"I'm sorry that you didn't get a letter. Maybe tomorrow you'll get one," said Jane as she handed her own to Molly.

"The return address says that it's from Lincolnville," said Molly.

"It must be from my mother. Please read it!" pleaded Jane.

"Dear Jane," Molly read, "I hope that you are well. We are fine here. Pop has been out working in the fields, and I've been doing a lot of sewing. Irma and Ruth have both gotten taller and I've had to make new dresses for them. I imagine that you're getting taller, too. You can try on some of Irma's clothes when you come home. If they don't fit, I'll make you something over Thanksgiving. I'm glad that you like learning Braille. I want to learn how to read and write it, too. Then I can write you letters, and you won't have to find someone to read my letters to you. Won't that be wonderful! It's time to feed the chickens. I'll write again soon. Love, Mother."

"Oh! I can't wait until Mom learns how to write Braille. Then I can read and re-read her letters whenever I want. But it takes a long time to learn Braille. Oh well. Maybe she'll be faster than me. Thanks, Molly, for reading my letter to me."

The excitement of learning Braille didn't stop the days from passing slowly that fall.

Even though Jane was happy to be learning new skills, she was still very homesick. Weekends were especially difficult. Many students went home, but the farm was too far away and train tickets too expensive for Jane to go home. Her best friend, Marie, became so homesick that her parents came to the school and took her home permanently. Jane was devastated. Now who would be her friend? Who else could understand her homesickness? Jane wrote letters and begged her parents to come and get her, but they never did.

Finally, it was November, and Thanksgiving was near. Charles took the train from Wabash to Indianapolis and brought her back for a short vacation at home. Jane was happy to be back with her family again, reveling in their attention. Everyone wanted to know what it was like at the school. Jane talked excitedly about her roommates, her nice teacher, and learning Braille. After months of bland institutional cooking, Thanksgiving dinner tasted especially good.

Yet, from the moment she arrived home, Jane dreaded the return to school. She kept busy chatting and playing with her sisters, willing herself not to think about leaving home again. All too soon, it was time to leave for the station.

"Mom, I don't want to go back to school," Jane said as tears slid down her cheeks. "I know that I need to go, but I miss you so much. And now that Marie isn't coming back, I don't even have my best friend."

"Now, Jane. Quit your crying. You'll be just fine. You made it to Thanksgiving, and it's only about three more weeks until you'll be back for Christmas," said Bessie, handing her a cotton handkerchief.

Not wanting to talk back to her mother but feeling misunderstood—three weeks was a long time—Jane fought to hold back the tears. Yet the harder she tried, the louder she sobbed.

Bessie gave her a long bear hug and said, "I love you. You've grown up so much just since September. I know that you'll be fine. Now it's time for you to go with Pop to the train station." She gave Jane a final squeeze and helped put on her heavy winter coat.

"Write lots of letters, Mom! And Ruth and Irma, send me letters too. I need lots of mail," Jane called as she turned to walk out the door.

In early January 1924, her teacher, Miss Jenkins, asked Jane to stop at her desk after class. "Jane, you've learned Braille very quickly. You know too much for this class. I think that it's time for you to move up to the fourth grade."

"But I'm not sure that I'm ready to move up," Jane blurted out. She was stunned that she'd have to meet other students and get used to a new teacher so soon after entering the school. Learning her way around another classroom was yet another adjustment that frightened Jane.

"Don't worry, Jane. I know that you can handle the work. You will start the fourth grade with Miss Stephens on Monday."

After spending the weekend worrying about her new teacher— would she be as nice as Miss Jenkins? —and how hard fourth grade might be, Jane walked through the crowded hall past her old classroom to her new room.

Miss Stephens was waiting for her. "Hello, Ella Jane. Welcome to fourth grade. Your seat is on the left side. Can you see the empty desk?"

Jane squinted and nodded, still cringing from hearing her full name. She'd always hated the name Ella and much preferred to be called Jane. She resolved to tell Miss Stephens after class. She was afraid that her new classmates would call her Ella Jane. That would not be a good way to begin fourth grade.

Heart pounding, Jane slowly made her way to her new desk. Even with little vision, she could feel all eyes of the other students upon her. A new girl in the class was a big event, and everyone in the fourth grade was curious about her.

Across the aisle from Jane sat a tall, thin boy named Mario Pieroni. A quiet and studious child, he was also curious about the new girl. Mario had no vision but relied upon his acute hearing to help him learn about her, listening closely when Jane answered a question. Her answers were thoughtful and intelligent. It didn't take long for him to decide that he liked the sound of her voice.

On a cold February morning, Jane waited to recite her memorized poem. Some children sputtered and couldn't remember the lines. Jane's heart beat faster as she listened.

"Jane, please stand and recite your verse," said Miss Stephens.

Trembling, Jane rose out of her chair and stood beside her desk. She was so close to Mario that he could have reached out and touched her, but of course he obeyed the rules. He listened with rapt attention as her wavering voice spoke the lines:

Today
Thomas Carlyle

So here hath been dawning Another blue Day:
Think wilt thou let it Slip useless away.
Out of Eternity
This new Day is born; Into Eternity,
At night, will return.

The moment she finished, Jane dropped into her chair and heaved a sigh of relief. She hated reciting in front of the class and was glad that the ordeal was over.

Little did she realize the effect the sound of her voice had on the boy across the aisle. Mario listened intently and memorized the poem as she recited the lines, later replaying her words countless times in his head as her voice echoed in his ears. He wished that he could congratulate her on her achievement, but the rules in 1925 against interactions between the sexes were unbending. He didn't want to get in trouble with the teacher if he talked to Jane. But the rules didn't stop him from thinking about her.

THE END OF SIGHT

SHORTLY AFTER JANE arrived at the school, the assistant governess insisted that Jane see the eye doctor who came monthly to examine students. The woman hoped that Dr. Morrison could do something to stop the glaucoma, but Jane did not expect a miracle. She knew that there was no cure.

The examination was short. The doctor sat back and said, "There's nothing that I can do. I'm sorry, Ella Jane."

"Yes, sir. Thank you, Dr. Morrison," said Jane. Even though she was only ten years old, she had become used to the idea of one day becoming totally blind and was not surprised that the doctor couldn't help her. She had expected that the visit would be a waste of time; her family doctor had said when she was born that there was no cure and for her parents not to waste their money searching for one. At least now the governess seemed assured that nothing could be done, and Jane would not be subjected to any further eye examinations.

Jane's vision continued to decline. She didn't want to complain about her constant headaches. She would be sent up to the third floor, where sick children were taken, to little rooms with nothing to do and no one to keep her company. The threat of being alone in the claustrophobic rooms was enough to keep her silent.

Jane's dorm room overlooked busy Meridian Street in downtown Indianapolis. Outside her window was a tall neon sign that seemed three stories high. She couldn't see the letters of what it advertised, but she loved to lie in bed at night and watch as it changed colors. It flashed a bright white light, then red, then green. The sign went dark, but a second or two later, came on again, repeating the cycle. The colors were pretty and helped relax her to fall asleep.

One clear night in April, Jane lay in her bed watching the lights. With a start, she realized that she couldn't see the red or the green flashes. She could see the blur of the white light, but not the colors. It was the last time she remembered seeing anything.

She wasn't sad to lose her sight; she just gave up. The next morning, she told Miss Black that she couldn't see. The governess didn't give any comfort to the girl, nor treat her any differently. Jane told herself that it really didn't matter, so she got dressed and went to school.

She was eleven years old.

:.

MARIO

IT WAS DAMP and foggy the day Mario was born in January 1914. The *Muncie Evening Press* reported, "The atmosphere was comparatively mild but very heavy." Physicians warned the public that the weather in Muncie, Indiana, was "very unhealthy and there are more cases of coughs, colds and lagrippe in the city than there have been for a long time."

But Eletta Pieroni wasn't worried about the weather or catching a cold. She was lying in her bed, holding her newborn son, her smile fading as she stared at his eyes.

"Antonio!" she said to her husband. "Look at his eyes! They are too big!"

"What? There's nothing wrong with his eyes," he said, peering over Eletta's arms for a better look at the baby's face. "He's just crying hard. His eyes are fine."

Eletta knew that Antonio was placating her. He couldn't help but notice that their baby's eyes were grossly enlarged, and while she understood that Antonio didn't want her to be upset after giving birth to their second child, she knew something was terribly wrong. Eletta looked at the doctor who had delivered her son. He shrugged and admitted, "I don't know if there's a problem. Maybe the swelling will go down. Let's just wait and see. But right now, I can't do anything for his eyes. I'm sorry."

Months later, another doctor diagnosed Mario with congenital glaucoma. The doctor explained that there was too much pressure in the baby's eyes, which damaged both optic nerves. Although he still had some vision, there was no treatment. One day, their child would be totally blind.

Stunned by the prognosis, Italian immigrants Eletta and Antonio worried about how they would raise a blind child. They would have to watch him constantly to ensure that he didn't hurt himself. Eletta, who spoke limited English, was already busy with three-year-old Charles and running the household. Antonio worked twelve-hour days at his downtown confectionery store, making and selling ice cream and candy. The store made enough money to support his family, but they lived simply and had no luxuries. The additional stress of coping with Mario's blindness and the expense of extra doctor visits added to the tension for both parents.

Besides trying to keep him safe, Eletta wondered if he could be educated. A blind child couldn't read or write. As faithful Catholics, both parents assumed that their children would attend their neighborhood parochial school, St. Lawrence. But now their baby would never be able to go to school. Eletta visualized a future where all Mario could do was to sit all day and wait for someone to entertain him. That picture terrified her.

Eletta and Antonio had many conversations about Mario's future. Antonio was worried that Mario would always be financially dependent upon him. Nobody would hire a blind man. What would happen to Mario when they died? Where would he live? Who would take care of him?

Yet, Eletta did not want to give up hope for a cure. Both Eletta and Antonio were devout Catholics and attended daily Mass. At home, they prayed at their shrine to the Virgin Mary for a miracle. In letters back to Italy, Eletta enlisted all family members to pray for Mario's healing. She was certain that God would answer her prayers.

The wood-framed family home was built south of downtown, across the street from busy railroad tracks. Coal was used to heat most buildings in 1917, and coal trains frequently traveled through Muncie on their way to Chicago. The steam engine's whistle alerted three-year-old Mario that a train was coming. He rushed to the porch and even in the coldest weather stood to watch the train's arrival just a couple of hundred yards away. The coal cars, loaded so that the coal was higher in the middle, were often topped with snow. Squinting his eyes, Mario could see the contrast between the black coal and white snow, thrilling him with the excitement of seeing the train and hearing the clacking of the wheels as it roared down the tracks.

Mario loved anything that moved: trains, the interurban, cars, and noisy trucks. He'd never been on a train or interurban and liked to imagine what it would be like to ride on one. What would it feel like to go so fast? How loud would the whistle be? The train whistles from across the street were loud enough to hurt his ears; he wondered how loud it would be if he was riding inside the car.

Early on a summer morning when Mario was three and a half, Eletta said to him, "Mario, we're going to take the interurban to Indianapolis today."

Mario stopped playing with Charles' (whom he called Charlie), wood blocks and jumped up to hug his mother. "Really? I can't wait! I've always wanted to go for a ride on the interurban."

"Today you are going to see a special eye doctor. Dad and I think that he can help you."

The prospect of riding on the interurban with his parents was exciting, almost making up for the pain he knew that he'd experience when the doctor probed his eyes.

Hoping for a miracle, the family boarded the interurban in Muncie and began their hour-long ride to the capitol city. Mario sat on his knees with his hands on the window to balance him. He smiled as he felt the air blow through the window, buffeting his face and mussing his hair. He could only see blurry shapes as the interurban passed farmhouses and barns, but he was enthralled with the constantly changing shapes and colors. The time passed quickly, and Mario was surprised when the railcar came to a stop at the station in downtown Indianapolis.

"Mario, we're here. We must get off now. Here, take my hand," said Eletta.

"But Mom, I want to keep going! I love the interurban."

"Remember that we'll ride it again after we see the doctor. That ride will be even better because then we'll be home again!" said Eletta.

After examining the young child, the doctor turned to Eletta and Antonio and said the words they wanted to hear. "I think that I can help Mario. I can do a surgical procedure which should relieve the pressure on his optic nerves. If the pressure is gone, then I think that he should regain some of his sight."

They readily agreed and with much hope arranged to have the surgery performed the following month.

But the surgery was botched. What limited vision Mario had before the operation was gone. He was left with nominal light perception—he could tell if the sun was out but couldn't actually see the sun. Now he could only hear the coal trains as their wheels clacked rhythmically on the tracks by his home. Mario cried and whimpered in pain for days after the surgery. He never forgot the agony and never forgave the surgeon for taking away what was left of his vision.

Mario wished that his parents would give up their search for a cure. He didn't mind being blind. He was happy playing with Charlie, who included him in games with his friends and taught him the names of neighborhood streets. Mario would grow to memorize the name and direction of almost every street in Muncie, and as a child, was proud to be able to walk alone without getting lost.

Eletta, perhaps feeling guilty about the failed surgery and becoming more desperate for a cure, took Mario to still more doctors. The only thing they could do was to give him eye drops, which stung his tender eyes. Mario squirmed and tried to resist the eye drops but was held down and forced to endure the pain. The drops did nothing to improve his sight.

As Mario's right eye swelled with the mounting pressure, the pain increased. It was especially agonizing at night, when his mother would hold him and softly sing Italian folk songs. While it soothed him, it didn't stop the pain.

Lying in bed in the room that he shared with his seven-year-old brother, Mario often distracted himself by listening to the trains as they passed by.

"Charlie, where do you think that train is going? What's in those big boxcars?" "Mario, how do you know that they're boxcars?"

"Oh, by the sound. Can't you tell the difference between a boxcar and a coal car?"

"No. I don't know how you do it." Charlie peered out the window. "Mario, you're right.

They're all boxcars. Maybe they're going to Minneapolis or somewhere in Canada."

"That would be exciting. Wouldn't it be fun to ride on a freight train, just to see where we'd end up?"

"I'd rather go on a nice passenger train. Let's go to sleep," said Charlie.

Mario tried to get comfortable under the blankets, but his eye hurt no matter if he lay on his back or side. He could tell by the sound of Charlie's breathing that he was already asleep and wished that his eye would allow him to sleep. Mario quietly counted the chimes of the living room clock as it rang eleven times. While trying to imagine himself as the engineer driving a huge steam engine, Mario finally fell into a troubled sleep.

But late one night when Mario was almost five, he couldn't keep the pain away by listening to trains or fantasizing about driving a big train engine. It became unbearable. He abruptly sat up in bed and touched his right eye just as it exploded. He was horrified to feel moist bits of his eye sliding down his cheek. He screamed in terror. Charlie woke up and tried not to vomit as he yelled, "Mom! Dad! Mario's eye burst!"

Mario felt Charlie's shaking hands grab his. "Mario! Don't touch your eye." Mario, feeling nauseated himself, didn't fight his brother.

Eletta and Antonio rushed into the room and turned on the light.

"Dio Mio! My God!" He heard his mother gasp and felt her handkerchief gently wipe his face. She pulled another handkerchief out of her pocket and held it softly against his eye, then sat down on his bed and enfolded him in her safe arms. Trembling and moaning, Mario heard his mother and father's voices arguing about calling a doctor, but what could a doctor do? His father said that no medicine could help a burst eyeball. His mother sighed and softly began praying in Italian.

Comforted by his mother's prayers, Mario calmed and began to relax. Suddenly, he realized that he had no more pain. "Mama!" he said. "My eye doesn't hurt anymore!"

She squeezed his hand. "Oh, Mario. Thank you, God, for that blessing."

Mother and son held each other tightly until the four-year-old fell asleep at last. The pain was gone, but so was his eye.

Months later, Eletta took him on a train to Cincinnati, hoping to find a doctor there that could cure his remaining eye. Again, she was unsuccessful. Just the thought of her son being totally blind for life was enough to keep her hoping and searching for someone, anyone, who could help. Prayer helped her get through each day, but so far hadn't produced her longed-for miracle. There was one other possibility of hope: an Italian faith healer who lived in the mountains not far from her home village of San Pietro. Perhaps she would be the one to cure her son.

ITALY

BY 1919, THE First World War was over, and it was finally safe
to travel to Europe. Eletta was anxious to return to Italy. She'd been
away from her family for over nine years and wanted her sons to
meet their Italian relatives. Even more importantly, she still hoped to
find someone to cure Mario's glaucoma. Eletta continued to pray for
a miracle and thought that if no one in America could help, surely
Italy would have the right doctor.

Mario was five and Charlie eight when they began the journey
to San Pietro in Campo. In preparation for the trip, Eletta had taken
a map of the United States and shown Mario the train's route. She
had gently taken his fingers and traced the route on the map from
Muncie to Cleveland, then northeast to Buffalo, east to Albany and
south along the Hudson River to New York City. Mario wanted to
know the names of all the cities and towns along the route, along with
questions about rivers and mountains that they would pass.

"Mom, I understand how we'll get to New York. But where is
Italy? How long will it take to cross the ocean? How big is the ocean?"
asked Mario.

"Mario! So many questions! The ocean is very big. It will take
us about ten days to cross it. Italy is on the other side of the ocean."

"How does the ship know where to go? If the ocean is so big, won't we get lost?"

Eletta smiled. "The ship has a captain. He knows how to steer the ship using a compass." "I know what that is. It shows which direction you're going. But where is Italy? The ocean is very big, isn't it? Could you show me on a map, like you did for the train?"

"We don't have a map of the ocean. Maybe we should go to the library. They have a globe, and I can show you the ocean. I'll put your fingers on New York, and then you can feel how big the ocean is to Italy. I can even show you where we'll get off the ship in Genoa."

"Mom! I'd love to do that. Can we go right now?"

Plans were made for Eletta and the boys to travel via train to New York City, then board the steamship *Re d'Italia* for Genoa. Antonio was sorry that he couldn't travel with them; he couldn't leave the store for an extended period. In 1919, ladies didn't travel alone or without a male escort. They were to be accompanied by their husbands, and until World War I, U.S. passports were issued as "Mr. Antonio Pieroni and wife." Eletta had her own passport; although she could legally travel alone with her children, societal rules insisted that she have a male escort for protection. Antonio's brother, Faust, agreed to accompany the family to New York City.

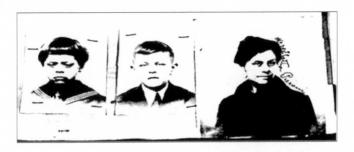

Passport photos: Mario, Charles, Eletta

Mario waited impatiently for Charlie's school to let out for the summer. Finally, on a warm, late June day, the family said a tearful goodbye to Antonio and boarded a train to Cleveland, where they would change trains for New York. While he could hardly wait to begin the trip, Mario's excitement was tempered by sadness that he wouldn't see his father again until the following summer.

Antonio and Faust watched as the porter loaded the heavy trunk and suitcases into the baggage car. The steam whistle blew a warning signal, and the conductor called, "All aboard!" Faust climbed up the steps into the second-class car and sat on the cloth seat next to Charlie. The boys waved from the open window, then sat back as the train slowly chugged away from the station.

The next day, they arrived in Cleveland, where they had a four-hour layover. To pass the time, Eletta and Faust took the boys to a nearby park next to Lake Erie. Tired from running and throwing stones into the lake, Mario asked, "Uncle Faust, why do we have to wait so long?"

"The next train to New York is only a first-class train. We don't have tickets for that one because it costs too much. We have to wait until the next train that has both first and second classes."

"Oh. Well, I wish that it would hurry up. I want to get on the boat!"

After spending two days sitting upright on an increasingly uncomfortable train seat, they finally arrived in New York. Faust loaded their luggage into a taxi and directed the driver to the dock where the ship, the *Re d'Italia*, was berthed. The steamship had only first and third classes. The third class was in steerage—a dark and unpleasant way to cross the Atlantic. Eletta chose the extra expense of traveling first-class to enjoy the fresh air and better accommodations.

When the captain noticed that she was traveling alone with two children, he invited the family to sit at the head table with him and his officers. Mario liked the extra attention from the staff, especially when the captain gave him chewing gum and candy.

Compared to other ocean-going ships, the *Re d'Italia* was small. But it was huge to Mario. The boys spent most of their time at sea roaming the first-class decks, exploring every nook and cranny. Eletta warned them not to go down to steerage, so of course they were curious to see the forbidden zone. Late in the afternoon of the second day at sea, Charlie decided that it wouldn't hurt to sneak down the stairs and see what was happening in steerage.

"C'mon, Mario! Let's go see what's down these steps!"

"But Mom said not to go down there," replied Mario.

"We won't tell her. And besides, we'll be quick. I'll tell you what I see."

Mario followed Charlie, both boys tiptoeing quietly as they descended into the darkness of the third-class deck. Charlie peered around the corner.

"Mario!" he whispered. "You won't believe this! There's a group of five men, and they're all eating out of the same big pot. With their hands! They're pulling out big gobs of spaghetti and eating it. They don't have any plates or forks!" As his eyes got used to the dark, he realized that everyone in the dining hall was grabbing the pasta with their hands and eating it hungrily. "Let's get out of here!" he said, and the boys ran back up the stairs, no longer worried about being quiet. With a new appreciation for their travel accommodations, they ran to the first-class dining room and joined their mother at the captain's table.

During the twelve-day journey, Mario learned to keep his balance as the ship pushed through the waves. He planted his feet wide apart while standing and reached for the handrails. He especially liked it when a wave lifted the ship up, then forced it down, smacking the water and making a huge splash. Sometimes water sprayed up onto his face, making him laugh with delight. Mario loved the motion of the ship and luckily never got seasick.

The brothers made friends with the sailors, asking questions about their jobs and learning about the big steam engines that propelled the boat. Mario listened for the engines' rumble and often put his hands on a wall or railing to feel the vibrations.

"Charlie! Come here and put your hands next to mine. Feel the engines? They're so strong that they make the walls shake! I can tell when the captain makes the ship go faster. The engines get really loud, and sometimes I think that the ship will fall apart!"

A nearby sailor overheard Mario's concern and said, "Don't worry, boy. This ship is very strong. But you're right, when we crank her up, she gets pretty loud."

"Well, I can't swim, so this ship had better not come apart and sink!" replied Mario.

The sailor smiled and said, "I've been on this ship for five years. She'll be afloat for a very long time."

When he wasn't following Charlie on explorations, Mario liked relaxing in a deck chair, feeling the sun on his face and wind whipping his hair. He breathed in the fresh air and tried to imagine the endless blue of the ocean. The squawk of a large seabird caught his attention.

"Charlie? I think that I just heard a bird! What's a bird doing out in the middle of the ocean?"

"It's flying around."

"Yes, but what happens when it gets tired? There aren't any trees. I thought that all birds live in trees."

"The bird just landed in the ocean. It's floating on the waves. Maybe it can sleep while it floats. Oh! It just dove under the water."

"Why would it do that, Charlie?"

"Maybe it's fishing. It must like fish. There's no dirt, so there aren't any worms like we have in Muncie."

"I miss the singing of the cardinals and robins at home. I love the sounds they make. How big is the bird?"

"A lot bigger than a cardinal. It's got really big wings. I think that it could fly a long way!"

After almost 2,500 miles, the ship made its first stop in the Azores Islands to refuel. Mario was fascinated by the idea of a speck of land in what felt like the middle of the huge Atlantic Ocean. He remembered that his mom had shown him the globe and put his fingers on the Azores. The islands had seemed very, very small compared to all the water around them. He wondered how the islands got there and what it would be like to live on an island. Where did the residents get their food? Mario knew about farms and wondered if the Azores had farms with corn or cows.

After being confined for days on the ship, Mario and Charlie happily ran ahead of their mother on the walk into town. The stop was a short one, with only enough time to explore the town and have lunch. The Azores had been of great strategic importance during the War when the United States had established a large naval base to aid Europe's defense. The Red Cross operated a restaurant and store to serve troops stationed on the islands. The restaurant was open to the public, so the family had lunch and dessert there, savoring their first ice cream since leaving Muncie. Mario wished that he had more time to explore the island. He wanted answers to his questions, but neither his mother nor Charlie seemed to have them. Someday he'd learn to read, just like his brother. Then he could learn about all the islands in the world by himself.

The next stop was Gibraltar, where the ship again refueled. The family disembarked and used the time to explore the Rock of Gibraltar and its famous limestone caves. Back outside in the bright sunlight, they went to the beach, where Mario enjoyed the seagulls' screeching and played chase with Charlie in the sand. All too soon, it was time to embark on the next leg of the journey to Naples.

The ship docked in Naples in the early morning five days later, which allowed the passengers a full day to tour. Eletta and a female friend she'd met on board decided that it would be enough time to take a side trip to Pompeii. The ancient city destroyed by the eruption of Mount Vesuvius was only seventeen miles away, and Eletta thought that it would be a good outing for the boys. After a full day of touring, they returned to the docks only to find an empty spot where the *Re d'Italia* should have been.

"Mio Dio," Eletta muttered under her breath. The two women became very upset as they realized that they had been left behind. Mario gripped his mother's hand tightly and struggled to understand what was going on.

"Mom, where's the ship?" asked Charlie.

"I don't know. Stay here. I'll go ask someone," she said as she released Mario's hand and hurried off towards a group of workers.

Mario listened as the tapping of her footsteps grew softer. Where was she going? Where was the boat? What was happening? His heart began to race, and he reached for Charlie's hand. Moments later, he heard her speak in rapid fire Italian and the equally fast replies from the men.

Eletta came running toward them, panting and out of breath. "Mario! Charles! Come with me! We need to find a telegraph office quickly. I have to tell my brother that we missed the boat!"

"Why Mom? What's going on? Can't we just telephone him?" asked Charles. "There are no telephones yet in Italy. The ship has left without us. I need to let Uncle Rocco know what happened, and the only way to do that is to send a telegram."

Shortly after sending the message, the group found the train station and managed to get tickets on a train to Rome. Although their ultimate destination was Genoa, it was the only train available that evening. Eletta was frantic; she worried that her brother wouldn't get the telegram and arrive at the docks, only to wonder why they weren't on the ship. All of their luggage was still aboard. The women had only their purses.

Arriving in Rome after midnight with two tired children, the women began searching for a place to sleep. After wandering around the darkened streets of downtown Rome, they asked a gentleman passing by if he could recommend a hotel. He gave them directions to a nearby rooming house; the women were quite relieved when the owner opened the door and said that she had one room available. After Eletta checked for bedbugs, all four of them piled onto the one bed and quickly fell asleep.

Early next morning, still wearing the same clothes from the day before, the weary group boarded the train to Genoa. While Mario enjoyed the ride, Eletta was anxiously looking at her watch, willing the train to go faster. When they finally pulled into the Genoa station, Eletta heaved a sigh of relief. While disembarking, Eletta said goodbye to her friend and heard her older brother calling her name.

"He's here! Come, children. Let's meet your Uncle Rocco," she said as she steered the boys toward the priest.

The brother and sister hugged and kissed each other on both cheeks, speaking Italian so fast that Mario couldn't understand their words. But he could tell that his mother was very happy to see her older brother, and suddenly, her mood felt lighter. Mario, too, began to relax. Rocco bent down and solemnly shook each boy's hand; suddenly laughing, he gave each a big hug, saying how pleased he was to meet them.

After the joyous reunion, they walked to the wharves where the *Re d'Italia* was already moored. The captain rushed down the gangway to meet them, apologizing profusely for leaving them in Naples. He'd waited for fifteen minutes but had to leave without them; apparently Signora Pieroni had misunderstood the departure time. Eletta was too tired and relieved to argue. She collected their belongings from the ship, and Rocco helped load the trunk into a horse-drawn cart for the short trip to the train station.

After a frightening journey from Naples to Genoa, Eletta was ready to relax on the five- hour trip to Barga, the town closest to San Pietro. Since it was a hot summer day, every window in the crowded train car was open. Mario leaned against his mother while Charlie napped across the aisle next to his uncle.

The wood-burning steam engine struggled to pull the long train uphill through the mountains. About halfway through one lengthy and very dark tunnel, the train jerked to a stop. Passengers began asking each other what was happening, but of course everyone was literally in the dark. There were no lights in the tunnel or the car. Men lit matches for a momentary glimpse of light, trying to ascertain why they were stopped.

Thick, acrid smoke from the engine drifted in through the open windows, and people began coughing. As the smoke filled the car, Mario reached for the handkerchief in his pocket and put it to his nose; it was little protection from the choking air. He felt his mother reach for his free hand. She was trembling and could offer little comfort. His eyes watered, but he was unperturbed by the dark. He was getting hot, though, and breathing was becoming harder.

Soon Eletta began praying quietly in Italian. Other women joined her; some voices were tinged with panic. At the same time, men shouted and cursed angrily, demanding to know why they were stopped. As there was no way to communicate with the train's engineer, the passengers had no choice but to sit and wait in the smoky darkness.

The prayers were comforting to Eletta, but she felt completely helpless in the hot, smoky air. It was pitch black, except for the occasional match that was lit and flickered for a few seconds. She called out to Charles and Rocco, asking if they were using their handkerchiefs.

Their muffled answers assured her that they were trying to filter the air. Passengers were coughing, trying to breathe. Some were waving their hands in front of their faces; others had newspapers to fan themselves.

Finally, after several hours, the passengers felt a bump as the engine connected with the car's coupler. The train started up, and minutes later, cleared the tunnel. Everyone cheered and clapped as fresh air flowed into the car and sunlight bathed the relieved passengers. Later, Eletta learned that the train was too heavy for the engine, so the engineer uncoupled part of the train and left it behind while he took the front to the closest station and parked those cars on a sidetrack. Then he backed the engine slowly down the tracks to pick up the remaining stranded cars in the tunnel.

After the harrowing experience, the family was exhausted but happy to be met at the station in Barga by Mario's paternal grand-mother, Umiliana Pieroni.

"Eletta! Carlo! Mario!" she called to them, smiling and waving, as she hurried to them. After a long, joyful hug with Eletta, she squeezed Charlie and pinched his cheeks; then Umiliana squatted down and looked carefully at Mario's eyes. She winced slightly at his enlarged eye and empty socket but said nothing.

"Il mio bambino! My baby!" she said while hugging him tightly. Caught up in her arms, Mario smelled the clean scent of Italian herbs. Her thin body felt soft and strong at the same time. Her arm muscles were strong from physical labor, yet he sensed a softness that radiated with love. When she took his hands, he felt the rough, calloused hands of someone who worked hard and was surprised that they felt even rougher than his mother's hands.

Umiliana had borrowed a donkey and a two-wheeled cart to take them up to her village, San Pietro in Campo. With the steamer trunk and luggage loaded into the cart, there was just enough space for Eletta and the children.

"Come! Let's go home. I know that you are all tired. Climb up and get as comfortable as you can," said Umiliana as she held on to the donkey's bridle.

Mario sat next to his mother, leaning up against her tense body and feeling the cart sway over the rough dirt road. He listened to the clopping of the donkey's hooves as Umiliana led the donkey back to the village, a two-hour ride that was mostly uphill. After a while, he felt his mother begin to relax as they approached familiar surroundings. The rhythmic motion of the cart lulled Mario into a nap, which ended when the cart came to a stop at the family home in San Pietro.

"We're here! Mario, wake up! Charlie, help get the smaller bags!" Eletta said as she gathered her belongings and lifted her skirt to climb down. She was immediately enveloped in the arms of her sisters-in-law, Maria and Antonietta, crying and hugging in a joyful reunion.

Neighbors stopped their chores upon hearing the excited voices and came running to greet Eletta and meet her children. Charlie and Mario, tired of traveling and wanting to explore their new surroundings, tolerated the hugs and kisses until Charlie asked, "Mom! Can we go inside? We want to see our room!"

"Mario will stay with me in this house. There's not enough room for you to sleep here, so you'll have your own room in the rectory with your Uncle Rocco and Anna."

"Who's Anna? And where's the rectory?"

"Anna is your uncle's housekeeper. The rectory is part of an old monastery that is over one thousand years old! You'll like it, and besides, you are only going to sleep over there. I lived there before I married your father. See? It's just across the street. We'll be very close by."

"Ok, Mom. Can we go now?"

"Yes. Listen for the church bell. Do you see it up there in the steeple? When it rings six times, it will be time for dinner."

"Mario! Let's go see Grandma's house!" said Charlie, reaching for his brother's hand.

Together they ran in to the old stone house but stopped short just inside the door. "What's that smell?" asked Mario.

"Mario! You won't believe it, there are cows in here! And hay! Oh! And a pig, too!" "And manure! That's what I smell. Yuck! What are animals doing inside the house?" "I don't know, but it looks like a barn down here. Where does this door go?" Charlie asked as he opened the heavy, creaking wooden door. "There are a whole bunch of big barrels in here. It says 'vino' on the side, so that must mean wine. Mom told me that they make their own wine, and we get to help pick the grapes. And there are smaller barrels that say 'olio d'oliva.' I think that's olive oil. Come here, you can touch the barrels to see the difference."

"It's cool down here and I can't feel any sun. There must not be any windows," said Mario as he put his arms around the olive oil barrels. "These barrels aren't very big; let me see the other ones." Mario ran his fingers on the wood, carefully avoiding splinters. "These barrels are a lot bigger," he said as he tried to put his arms around the container. "I can't even get my arms around it. Grandma sure has a lot of wine. Do you think that they'll give us any?"

"No, silly, that's why they have cows. We have to drink milk. Let's get out of here!"

The boys ran up the stairs to the next level, where they found the main living area anchored by a kitchen and a large fireplace, which was used for cooking and also served to heat the eight-hundred-year-old house. There were two small bedrooms off to the side; they were rented out to a young widow, her daughter, and two sons. She and the children chopped wood, cared for the animals, plowed the fields, and harvested the crops in return for room and board.

After a cursory inspection of that level, Charlie and Mario went up to the next floor and found three bedrooms. Their aunts, Antonietta and Maria, shared one, Umiliana had the largest, and Mario and Eletta would share the third room. Each room was simply furnished; an iron bed stood next to a small wood table, and since there were no closets, there was a plain armoire against one wall. On the table stood two metal candlesticks with candles that had been burned down to short stubs. Simple pieces of white cloth served as curtains, covering the one tall, narrow window in the room. A crucifix of Jesus was displayed prominently on one wall of each room, an overt reminder of their Catholic faith.

"Charlie? Where's the toilet? We haven't found it yet," said Mario.

"It must be behind this door," Charlie answered as he opened it. "Yes, it's here. But it doesn't look like what we have at home!"

"It smells awful! Did somebody forget to flush it?"

"That's the thing. It's just got an old wood seat, but there's no water. And you can't flush it. Pee-you! It stinks."

"Well, how do you use it? Ewww. I'm going to hold it for a long time. It's awful in here."

"I see a pipe that goes down somewhere. Let's go see where it comes out!"

The boys ran down the flights of stairs while their grandmother watched with a smile. She knew that they'd discovered the primitive toilet and would soon be back with questions.

Minutes later, Charlie and Mario were back, looking confused.

"Grandma," said Charlie, "We looked everywhere but couldn't find that pipe! Where does it go?"

"Do you know what a cistern is?" she asked.

"We have one at home that holds water," said Charlie.

"There's a cistern under the house. The pipe goes down into it. Every year in the springtime, we take buckets and empty it out. Then we dump the buckets on the fields and spread it around for fertilizer. It helps makes everything grow, and, in the summer, we get delicious tomatoes. And next spring, you both will get to help with the buckets!"

Charlie looked at his grandmother in disbelief while Mario wrinkled his nose at the prospect of the dirty job.

Laughing, Umiliana looked down at her grandchildren and said, "Don't worry! Bucket season is a long way off. Go out now and find Charlie's bedroom at the monastery. Uncle Rocco will be waiting for you."

* * *

In September, after Charlie began third grade at the village school, Eletta took Mario to Florence, where a doctor examined him.

"I'm sorry, Signora Pieroni, but I'm afraid that young Mario has glaucoma. It's very rare to find glaucoma in a child this young," said Dr. Rizzo in Italian. "His optic nerve has been damaged, and there's nothing that I can do to fix it. The operation he had in the United States, even though done with the best of intentions, made things worse."

"Maybe you have some medicine that will help," said Eletta.

"There is no medicine, no eye drops, no operation that will bring back his vision. I know that the American doctors have tried many things. I wish that I could help."

Tears began rolling down her cheeks. Eletta struggled to comprehend that her worst fears were coming true. "You're saying that he'll be blind for his whole life! How do you know? Maybe there will be a miracle and one day he'll be able to see!"

Dr. Rizzo stood up and put one hand on her shoulder. "Signora Pieroni, you're right. We can always pray for a miracle. Meanwhile, take Mario home and allow him to be a boy. Let him do things that his brother does. Mario is a very bright boy. Make sure that he goes to school. He might surprise you."

Mario was not upset with the news that his eyes could not be fixed. He was happy that the doctor said not to waste more time or money on seeing other doctors and was especially relieved that he would not have to endure any more stinging eyedrops. He was ready to go on with his life, even if his mother was reluctant to accept the doctor's advice.

Smiling, Mario asked, "Mom? Can we go now? The doctor said that I don't need any medicines or eyedrops. I want to go home and play with Charlie."

Returning to San Pietro in Campo, Eletta was devastated but unwilling to give up on prayer, the only thing that gave her hope. She took Mario to the many roadside shrines in the area; most were statues of the Virgin Mary or beautiful icons painted of Mary and baby Jesus. The nearby town of Barga alone had ten shrines, which they visited, often taking flowers as an offering. They knelt before the statues, Mario fidgeting while his mother prayed for a miracle. He obediently waited for his mother to finish praying but couldn't wait to get back home to play with Charlie. His blindness didn't bother him; he didn't remember being able to see. It was just a fact of life. He wished that his mother wouldn't be so upset about him, but he didn't know how to comfort her.

When his eyes didn't change, Eletta decided to take him to a faith healer who had a reputation for helping believers. They walked up mountain trails a mile to the woman's home. Even though Mario enjoyed the time with his mother, he was silently dreading what the healer might do to him. He hoped that she wouldn't put anything that stung into his eyes.

Upon their arrival at the woman's home, she took him to a shed, where piles of chestnuts were being dried on the floor. Chestnuts were a favorite treat in Italy and were often roasted over the fireplace while neighbors gathered to enjoy each other's company and drink wine. Mario accidentally stepped on some, which produced a loud crunching sound and startled him. He was relieved when the woman said nothing.

She directed him to sit on a wood chair. Taking a crucifix from the wall, the woman handed it to him and said, "Hold this, child." Not knowing what she wanted him to hold, Mario obediently took the sacred object. Using his fingers to feel the object, he traced the body of Christ hanging from the cross and recognized it as a crucifix.

The healer placed her hands over the boy's eyes and began incanting a long prayer in a language that he didn't understand. She raised her voice, and then dropped it dramatically while murmuring repetitive phrases. Finally, after what seemed an eternity to the child, she stopped and removed her hands from his eyes.

Satisfied, she put her hands on his and looked at his eyes for confirmation of the miracle. "What can you see?" she asked.

"Nothing. Just a little light. Can we go now?"

Mario wasn't surprised that the woman didn't cure him. He felt a little embarrassed by all the attention; even though he was only six years old, he didn't have faith in the woman. His blindness didn't bother him—it only distressed his mother. He knew that his parents worried about him, but as long as he had Charlie, he was happy.

Distraught that her last resort was unsuccessful, Eletta continued to pray for a miracle. She wrote long letters to Antonio, telling him of her efforts and sadness that no one had been able to help their son. They wrote of their fears for their son's future: how would he make a living? She'd seen beggars on the streets in Florence. Would her son be a beggar? How could he go to school if he couldn't see to read? What would she do with him all day?

The parents decided to make any sacrifice necessary so that Mario would not want for anything when he grew up. Antonio vowed to work even longer hours to be a successful storeowner; Eletta promised to help by working there on Saturdays making pork tenderloin sandwiches and waiting on customers.

A year after arriving in Italy, the family returned to Muncie, and the new, larger home that Antonio had bought while they were gone. He'd turned the house into a duplex, renting out the upstairs. It was closer to the store than the previous house and provided a new neighborhood for the boys to explore.

Antonio and Eletta talked with Charlie, telling him that since Mario would never be able to see, he needed to look after his brother and include him in his play as much as possible. They wanted Mario to live a full life, and Charlie would play a key role. He would be responsible for Mario's safety. As a young boy, Charlie never imagined how much of an influence he would have on Mario's life. He accepted his role with verve and imagination, often leading his younger brother on adventures best not revealed to their parents.

.. :

MARIO GOES TO SCHOOL

ST. LAWRENCE CATHOLIC School, which Charles attended, refused to admit Mario to the first grade because he was blind. The principal didn't want to give special attention to one child, believing that it was unfair to the other children. She had no recommendations for alternative education and left the clear impression that it would be a waste of time to try to educate him. He could never earn a living, so why bother teaching him academic subjects?

However, perhaps feeling obliged to save his soul, the principal agreed that Mario could attend school only for catechism class. Charles would walk with him to school, and afterward, the teacher would assign a male classmate to walk him home.

But twice-weekly catechism class hardly made up for the long, lonely days that Mario spent wishing that he could go with Charlie to school. Every weekday, he followed his mother around the house bored with nothing to do. Eletta didn't think that he could help her do the chores and had no time to entertain or read to Mario. Mario missed his brother, often dogging Eletta and asking several times a day, "When will Charlie get home?"

The nun, who hadn't even interviewed Mario, thought that a blind child was impossible to educate. But Antonio and Eletta knew how quickly he learned and had seen his keen interest in the world around him. While dismayed at the principal's attitude, they became determined to help their son get an education.

Two years later, when Mario was eight years old, Antonio learned from a friend about the Indiana School for the Blind. Because it was fifty-five miles away in Indianapolis, Mario would need to stay in a dormitory during the week. Eletta was uncertain about her young son spending so much time away from home with strangers. He was only eight! She couldn't tuck him into bed at night, nor cook good Italian food for him. And what if he got sick? She couldn't take care of him. It pained her to think that he would be gone for days at a time, returning only on the weekends.

When Antonio and Eletta told their son about the school, he didn't understand the implications of living far from home, but jumped at the chance to learn reading and writing. Instinctively, Mario knew that it was time for him to get an education, even though it meant leaving home and his adored older brother. Mario had never met another blind child, and while he was happy playing with Charlie and his friends, he was excited to make new friends.

Very early on his first day of school in September 1922, Mario and Eletta walked to the interurban station and boarded the train. Eletta spoke little English and felt uncomfortable taking Mario by herself. Her friend, Mrs. Huffer, joined them on the train. She would help them find the school and get Mario settled. During the ride, Mrs. Huffer gave Mario a little gold ring with his initial *M* on it. He was very proud of it and kept it as a favorite lifelong possession.

Upon arrival at the school, Mrs. Huffer helped Eletta with the paperwork while Mario sat on a chair and anxiously swung his legs. The school smelled clean, like the floors had been mopped with bleach.

He wondered where the dining room was; he couldn't smell food cooking and he was getting hungry. He hoped that it wouldn't be long before lunch. His mother's soft voice echoed off the plaster ceiling and walls, telling him that he was in a large room. The school seemed like a very big place—much larger than anything that he'd experienced in Muncie. How would he ever find his way around? He shuddered as he pictured himself walking aimlessly alone through the long halls, not knowing where he was or how to find help.

Heavy footsteps came from his right. A deep male voice said, "Hello! Mrs. Pieroni? I'm Superintendent Wilson. I'm so pleased to meet you." Turning to Mario, who stood when the man announced himself, he continued, "And you must be Mario. Welcome to the Indiana School for the Blind." Mr. Wilson took Mario's hand and gently shook it.

"Thank you," said Mario.

"We're glad to have you with us, Mario. I know that you'll like it here. I bet that you'd like to see your room. Miss Johnson will be your governess. She will show you to your room. You'll have five roommates—all of them are nice boys your age. I'll let you get settled in now."

Mario held his mother's hand as they walked past classrooms, the dining hall, and the gym. He thought that he'd never find his way around this gigantic school. He was already lost. They'd walked down one long corridor, turned right, went down another hall, and up a wide flight of stairs. After he felt like they'd walked a mile, they finally arrived at his new room.

"Here we are, Mario. Your bed is over by the window. You have a chest of drawers next to it. That's where you'll keep your clothes," said the governess. "Your roommates aren't here right now, but you'll meet them soon. I'll let your mother and Mrs. Huffer help you get settled."

Eletta and Mrs. Huffer unpacked his suitcase and made up his bed while Mario stood by the open window listening to the distant sound of children's voices on the playground. He missed playing with Charlie and their friends in Muncie. He didn't know anybody at the school, and soon he'd be left all alone.

"Mario, come here," Eletta said. "I want you to see where I put your clothes." Mario followed the sound of her voice and lightly touched his bed as he walked obediently to his mother.

"Here's the top drawer. I put your underwear and socks in there." Mario dutifully put his hands in the drawer, feeling the soft fabrics and noting their location. "Your shirts are in the next

Drawer, and your pants are in the bottom drawer. You know how to dress yourself. They won't help you here with your bath or brushing your teeth."

"I know, Mom. I'm eight years old. I can take care of myself."

Eletta smiled at Mrs. Huffer. She knew that her son was strong-willed, but leaving him there in the care of strangers was almost unbearable. She dreaded saying goodbye, knowing that Mario would be upset when she had to leave. It would be hard to comfort him while choking back tears. She hesitated, looked around the room, and wondered how the governess managed to get all six boys to sleep. She hoped that Mario would make friends with them.

When there was nothing left for them to do, Eletta hugged her son tightly, and Mrs.

Huffer patted him on the head.

"Mom! Don't go," sobbed Mario as he reached for his mother. "Don't leave me here. I want to go back with you."

Eletta struggled to hold back her own tears. How could she leave behind her terrified, blind son with strangers? She began to waver.

Mrs. Huffer looked at her sternly and said, "Eletta, we need to go now, or we'll miss the train. Goodbye, Mario. I'm sure that you'll do just fine.

Your governess is here, and she'll help you."

"No! No! Oh Mom, please take me with you."

"Goodbye Mario. I'll see you on Friday. That's not far away." The women turned and left him in the care of the unknown governess, the sounds of his cries echoing down the institutional hallway.

While weekends home had seemed like a good compromise to Eletta, she hadn't anticipated the emotional costs involved. Every Friday, Mario got excited to come home. But every Monday morning was miserable for both parent and child. Mario cried inconsolably and begged his parents to not go back. When that didn't work, he complained that he was sick with a stomachache.

"Mom, I'm sick! I can't go back to school," said Mario with the appropriate moaning sounds meant to convince his mom that he needed to stay home.

Eletta had to decide quickly if his pain was real or if it was his imagination. She didn't want to miss the interurban. But what if he really was sick? She couldn't take him to school sick. Eletta touched his forehead.

"I don't think that you have a fever. I can't keep you home. We have to hurry now to get to the train," she said.

Disappointed, Mario picked up his small suitcase and put on his coat.

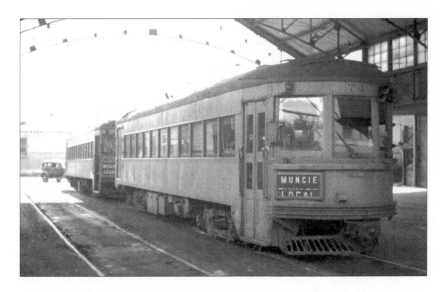

Interurban at the Muncie station. Photo courtesy of Jeff Koenker

The weekly ritual was exhausting to Eletta. Antonio complained that it was taking too big of a toll on her and Mario. It irked him that Eletta was spending so much on the train fares. Two round trip fares for two people every weekend was adding up. They decided to make a deal with Mario for second grade. For every weekend that he'd stay at school, they would put the train fare into a bank account for him. That was a big incentive for him to stay, and it turned out to be much easier emotionally since he didn't have the Monday morning tears upon leaving home. By the time he reached sixth grade, he didn't go home for weeks at a time.

The campus consisted of four buildings, and Mario was overwhelmed at first. There was no one to walk with him or guide him to class or even the bathroom. He was on his own. At home, he knew the names of every street in his neighborhood and which direction they went. But the campus was confusing until he asked a teacher which direction each building faced. Armed with that information, he oriented himself. Being aware of his location and the direction he was headed was key to not getting lost either in school or later as an adult traveling the streets of a big city.

In 1922, the students at the Indiana School for the Blind spent little time in their dorm rooms, using their rooms only for sleeping. They were required to stay downstairs in the sitting rooms when not in class. The sitting rooms were two adjoining rooms with tables and chairs. The governess or her assistants watched over the students as they read or played games, making sure that they behaved.

In good weather, they played outdoors. They spent hours on the playground swings and often teamed up to play a game called "Run Under." One child sat on the swing while another one pushed him up so high that he could run under him. The object for the child on the swing was to go as high as he possibly could. Mario loved to swing and feel the air in his face and hair. He imagined that he was flying, feeling a freedom that was impossible when he was on the ground.

As he got a little older, roller-skating became a popular activity. The grounds had extensive walkways that were perfect for skating, although the boys were limited to their side of the campus. They dared not cross the line over onto the girls' side, as contact between the sexes was strictly forbidden. Mario learned every bump, every inch of the sidewalks, and rarely fell. His noisy skate wheels rolled on concrete, creating echoes that bounced off the covered walkways and building walls. By listening carefully to the acoustics, he could tell if he was close to a building or under a walkway. Holding hands with a friend, they went in and out and around columns outside the main building. They felt fearless.

On a cold but sunny winter day, the noon lunch bell rang, signaling that it was time to line up for lunch in the dining room.

"Arthur," said Mario. "I want you, Melvin, and William to sit with me. We can plan what we'll do after school today."

The boys hesitated, unsure of what to say. Melvin and William, who had some vision, looked wistfully at each other while Arthur scuffed his shoe as he tried to think of a reply. Finally, Arthur said, "We can't sit with you. We sit over at another table in the corner."

"Why not? You just sit by yourselves in the corner? With nobody else?" asked Mario.

"We just have to sit there, that's all," said Melvin.

"Well, I don't understand why you can't sit with me. That's just plain dumb."

"Leave it alone, Mario. We're used to it. We have our own room, too. They don't want us in with the white boys."

Mario, who had never been exposed to racial prejudice, finally understood what they were trying to tell him. They couldn't sit together because of their skin color. Instinctively, he knew that was wrong, but since his friends seemed to accept the situation, he reluctantly accepted it as well.

After experiencing his mother's savory Italian cooking, Mario found it hard to stomach the plain institutional food. Breakfast was Corn Flakes and sometimes canned fruit. For lunch and dinner, there was often stringy beef with watery gravy, boiled potatoes, and canned fruit for dessert. The beef was difficult to eat. Cutting it took a lot of effort, especially with the dull knives given to the children. The thin gravy dripped on his shirt, no matter how hard he tried to avoid getting himself dirty. If he couldn't stomach the main course, he had a peanut butter sandwich. The cottony white bread at school was tasteless, but a peanut butter sandwich was better than being hungry. Nothing was as filling as his mother's warm, freshly baked bread. A wave of homesickness passed over him as he remembered the smell and taste of her bread.

Despite the unappetizing food and lack of fresh vegetables, Mario was healthy most of the time. But if he did catch a cold or didn't feel well, he didn't tell anyone; there were no doctors or nurses on staff. The standard treatment for any malady was a dose of "salts" administered by the governess. Getting a dose of Epsom salts in warm water was worse than the original illness, as it was a strong laxative. Mario suffered the consequences of one dose the first time he complained of a headache. He resolved not to complain again.

If someone became more seriously ill, he was taken to the top floor and put in isolation. That frightened Mario, as he couldn't think of anything worse than being stuck alone in a room with nothing to do but be sick. It reminded him of when he was four years old and sick with the flu during the 1918 influenza epidemic. Public health officials warned that the flu was extremely contagious and deadly, with thousands of people around the world dying every day. Despite it being February, Eletta had made a bed for him out on the cold sleeping porch. She was terrified that other family members would get sick. Although she tried her best to care for him, she was afraid to spend much time with her sick child. Sick with a fever and body aches, Mario hated being isolated on the porch with nobody to talk to or comfort him. He used his vivid imagination to entertain himself, since books were of no use to him, and radio broadcasts were not yet established. He missed running and playing with Charlie. For the two weeks it took him to recover, time moved very slowly in his dark world.

It wasn't surprising that when he contracted measles during the sixth grade at the School for the Blind, he panicked at the thought of being forced into a sick room and isolated. Based upon his experiences with the governess and her assistants, he knew that he'd receive only minimal care. He wanted to be at home, where his mother could take care of him.

Mario had a fever and could feel the raised bumps of the rash on his body. He knew that he needed to get home before the governess saw the rash or suspected that he was ill. He called his father at the store, who left immediately for Indianapolis and brought him home. As an adult, Mario sometimes wondered how many people he'd exposed on the train to the serious virus, but at the time, he wasn't concerned about others. He was relieved to be with his father and would soon be home in his mother's loving care. It would take two weeks for Mario to recover, but he was grateful to be in his own bed, reading Braille books to help pass the time.

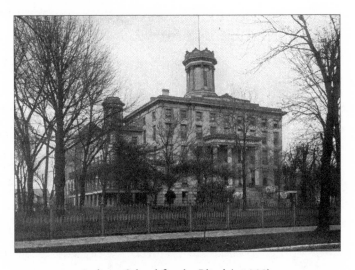

Indiana School for the Blind (c.1922)

ADVENTURES WITH
CHARLIE

THE NOISE OF the crane's engine—its grating gears and screeching metal—as it worked to lift heavy steel beams was exciting to Mario. It sounded powerful to the blind ten year old, who imagined the beams dangling in the air and caught by the men he heard yelling high above him. He'd played with his older brother's Erector Set, a construction set that allowed him to understand gears, beams, and pulleys. He'd felt the grooved edges of circular shapes and assembled long, narrow, metal beams with nuts and bolts. But standing yards away from the life- sized action was much more interesting than playing on the living room floor. He loved the sparking sound of the welders' torches as they connected beams to form another floor of the building. Turning his head in different directions changed the sound. He was never bored down at the construction site just a block away from his home on East Charles Street.

Topping out at three floors, the new YWCA seemed as tall as a skyscraper to Mario and his then thirteen-year-old brother. In the summer of 1924, the boys often stood on the sidewalk next to the site, their necks sore from straining to look up at the workers.

When the framework was finished in July, the steel girders resembled a jungle gym and gave Charlie an idea. "Hey Mario!" he said one evening. "Let's climb up to the top! I'll show you how this thing is built."

"But aren't there any workers here?"

"No. The workers are all gone for the day. We won't get caught."

Mario, who adored his older brother and never turned down an adventure with him, readily agreed to the ascent. He reached for his brother's elbow and lightly grasped it; the boys carefully made their way through construction debris to a ladder leaning against the building.

"I'll go first. Mario, you stay right behind me. It's pretty tall, maybe even sixteen feet!" said Charlie as he began to climb up the creaky wooden ladder.

"Okay. I'm coming," Mario said, reaching with his right hand for the next rung of the ladder. Concentrating on listening to his brother climb, Mario kept pace. Sweat trickled down his face, causing a tickle, but he didn't pause to wipe it away. He wanted to stay close to his brother. Soon, he heard Charlie stop and felt the ladder jiggle as Charlie dismounted.

"Alright, Mario. You're at the top of the ladder. Step to your right, and I'll make sure that you don't fall."

Mario extended his right foot, testing the wooden platform before putting his whole weight down. Charlie took his hand, steadying him, then said, "Good, now take my arm and we'll go to the next ladder."

"You mean we have another ladder to climb? I thought the first one would take us to the top."

"We have two more ladders if we want to get to the top. Remember? There are three floors. We have a lot more climbing to do." Charlie hesitated. "Are you afraid?"

"Oh no! I'm not scared. Show me the next one. I want to get to the top." Mario had no fear of falling. He felt safe, with complete trust in his brother.

"Okay, let's go. Follow me, just like you did before."

The boys continued their climb, the sun beating down on them that Saturday afternoon.

Mario again concentrated on listening to his brother's movements and was relieved when Charlie stopped for the last time. Charlie breathed heavily, both from the effort and the concentration on watching his brother. "Mario, we made it. We're at the top. Get off just the way you did before."

Concentrating on his instructions, Mario successfully dismounted and stood still to catch his breath. A warm breeze whistled through the structure. "Oh—that wind feels good. I'm hot from all that climbing. What do you see, Charlie?"

"Lots of beams that go in all different directions. And there are no walls or ceilings yet, so I can see lots of trees back toward our house. And there's downtown. I can see pretty far away."

"Now what are we going to do? Climb back down?"

"No, let's stay up here for a while. We should sit and rest."

"Okay, where do we sit? Are there any chairs?"

Charles chuckled. "There aren't any floors, so we'll just go sit on one of those beams."

"You mean, there's no place to walk except on a beam? How are we going to do that? And aren't we up awfully high? If I fall, there's no place for me to land."

"Well, you'd land in the basement. But don't worry, I won't let that happen. Now, let me show you how wide the beam is. Squat down and put your hand right here," said Charlie. He took Mario's hand and placed it on the warm beam.

He used both hands to explore the width and depth of the steel. "That's not very wide," he said. "It feels like it's only a few inches across. How are we going to walk on it?"

"We're not going to walk. We'll crawl on all fours. You put your left hand on my hip. I'll go slowly."

Mario did as he was told, working to maintain his balance with only one hand as he crawled along the narrow surface. Charlie stopped and said, "Let's sit here. This is a good place. I can see lots of buildings."

The boys slowly lowered their hips to the girder, then swung their legs over the side, laughing as their legs dangled in the air. Holding on tightly to the beam, Mario moved his head back and forth as he listened for sounds that were different at that height.

"I hear a train, Charlie! It sounds like a big freight engine. I bet that's a Nickle Plate train, way over near South Walnut Street. It's getting closer, so it must be moving pretty fast," said Mario. "What else can you see from up here?"

"I can see a long way," said Charlie. "There's the St. Lawrence Church steeple. It's tall and goes up to a point. There's a cross at the very top." Turning his head toward downtown, he said, "And I can see the Roberts Hotel. It's even bigger than this building will be. I'll count the number of stories. One, two, three, four, five, six. Wow. That's tall. I can see all the way down to the courthouse, too!"

Charlie wanted to show Mario exactly how high up they were and finally had an idea. "Mario, I want you to listen!" He hacked up a big glob of spit and let it loose.

After a long moment, Mario exclaimed, "I heard it! That's a long way down there! It must be in the basement!"

"That's how high up we are. Don't fall off, because you'll be down there with the spit!"

"I'll be careful," Mario said with a shudder, then coughed up his own spit and listened for the splat. Mario felt alive with the thrill of conquering the building. He was, quite literally, on top of his world.

"Mario, I'm getting hungry. Let's go down now."

Mario again placed his hand on his brother's hip and followed him slowly along the girder to the interior where the ladders were located. Climbing down was easier and faster than the ascent; they were home before supper, with their parents none the wiser.

They were not caught in the act, but word did get back to their father.

"Antonio, I tell you, those boys were at the very top! And Mario could have fallen off!" said their neighbor. "You're crazy to let your blind boy and Charlie climb around on that building."

Antonio was unfazed by the report. "Mario is safer than Charlie because he has to use all his wits to not fall. I won't tell him that he can't do something that his brother can do. How will he learn if he sits around the house all day?"

LESSONS

THE SUN BEAT down unmercifully on Mario, Charlie, and two neighbor boys. Tired of playing marbles on the sidewalk that was hot even in the shade, Charlie said, "Hey boys, let's go swimming in the old gravel pit."

"But I don't know how to swim," said Mario. "And besides, Dad said that it's dangerous to go down there. It's really deep, and he said there are No Trespassing signs. What if we get caught?"

"You're only ten years old. They won't do anything to you. They'll just tell us to go home," said Charles. "And remember you were worried about getting caught while we climbed up the YWCA. Nothing happened there, and more people could have seen us."

"I wish that we could just swim in White River. It's not deep," answered Mario.

"That river is really dirty. Nobody swims in it. The gravel pit isn't that deep. Come on, Mario, let's go. I'll teach you how to swim."

"But how will we get there? It's too hot to walk that far," complained Mario.

"I know a shortcut. Come, take my elbow and I'll show you. You love trains, don't you? We're going to take the railroad bridge over the river. Then it won't be a long walk, and we can go jump into that cool water!"

"The railroad bridge? You mean we'd walk on the train track over the river?" Although he and Charlie had walked many times on train tracks, he'd never attempted crossing a trestle over water. It sounded almost as scary as swimming in the forbidden gravel pit. "Charlie, what if a train comes when we're in the middle? We could all be killed!"

"Mario, quit worrying. I have a plan. We'll be fine. Let's go—I'm tired of being hot."

Trusting his beloved brother, Mario took Charlie's elbow, and the four boys set off on their adventure, walking several blocks to the tracks. Finding no trains, they walked between the rails on the wood ties until they approached the river. Ignoring the *No Trespassing* signs prominently displayed, the boys stopped at the edge of the trestle and waited for Charlie's directions.

"Mario, we're at the bridge. I don't hear any whistles, but I can't see very far away because there are curves on both sides. Here's what you'll do: We'll watch for trains, but you put your ear down on the track and listen. See if you can hear a train coming."

Obediently, Mario lay down on the rail and listened. Seconds later, hearing no rumbling train, Mario said, "I don't hear anything. There's no train coming."

"Let's go," said Charlie as he grabbed his brother's hand to help him up. The boys started crossing the river, stepping carefully on the ties; there were no railings to prevent them from falling thirty feet down into the river.

"I can see the water way down there, Mario," said Charlie, occasionally looking behind them for an approaching train.

Mario shuddered and was glad that he couldn't see how high up he was. *What if a train came along when they were in the middle of the trestle? What would I do?* he thought. Mario decided that he'd quickly stick his legs over the side and hang there until the train passed. He wasn't sure that would save him, but he could always jump off and into the water. He'd rather drown than get smashed by a steam engine.

Once across the river, they hiked about three miles to the gravel pit. They snuck under the rusty gate, ran to the water's edge, and stripped off their clothes. The older boys jumped in, squealing with delight at the freezing water.

"How deep is this pit? Is it still being mined?" asked Mario.

"No, this old pit hasn't been used in years. Nobody will catch us. And it's deep. Real deep! But don't worry. Come on, Mario. I'll teach you how to swim," said Charlie.

Mario had complete trust in his brother. He learned to put his face in the water and kick his feet. That lesson was the start of a lifelong love of swimming, something that Mario did whenever he had the chance.

* * *

Charlie began working at his father's confectionery store when he entered high school. Within a year, he saved enough money to buy a used jalopy, a 1921 Ford Touring car, for $15. In 1925, there was no minimum age for driving, and driver's licenses weren't invented yet, so Charlie taught himself to drive at age fifteen. Antonio wasn't interested in driving and never wanted a car, but he did insist that his son insure it for $20.

One summer afternoon, Charlie asked Mario if he'd like to go for a ride. Twelve-year-old Mario happily put down the Braille book he'd been reading and jumped out of his chair. "Let's go," he said.

"Do you want to drive?" Charlie asked.

Startled, but always up for a challenge, Mario replied, "Sure. But I don't know how to drive."

"Don't worry, I'll teach you. Come around to the driver's side," he said while opening the door. "It's lucky that this car is a convertible and we don't need the roof. You don't have to worry about banging your head. Now put your foot on this running board," said Charlie, tapping the metal so Mario could find it with his hands. Mario climbed up and settled into the driver's seat.

"I found the steering wheel," Mario said, feeling the warmth of the smooth wood as he ran his hands around the big circle. "How do I steer this thing?"

"It's easy. I'll stand behind you in the rumble seat so I can see everything. I'll tell you which way to turn by tapping on your shoulder. But first, I want to show you the pedals. The accelerator is by your right foot. Reach down and you can feel it. You push that with your foot. The harder you push, the faster we'll go."

"Now reach over to your left and feel the brake. It's up a little higher than the other one." "I found it. Let me practice with my feet." Mario used one foot for each pedal, experimenting with pressure needed to make the pedal move.

"Okay, now I'll start her up," Charlie said as the car roared to life. He hopped into the rumble seat behind Mario and put one hand on each of Mario's shoulders.

"Feel my right hand, Mario? If I want you to angle right, I'll push a little on your right shoulder. The same with going left. I'll push on your left shoulder. But if you need to make a sharp turn, I'll push down harder, like this."

Mario felt the unmistakable pressure of his brother's hand on his shoulder and yelled in pain. "Ow! You don't have to push that hard. You want me to turn right?" Mario practiced turning the wheel.

"I'll tell you how fast to go. When I want you to stop, I'll push down on both shoulders.

Ready?"

"Ready," Mario said, as he gingerly pushed down on the pedal and the car jerked forward. "Whoa. I'm driving!" His face alit with glee, he turned around to his brother and said, "Where are we going?"

"How about out in the country? It's a real pretty day. Go right up here at Main Street," directed Charlie as he gently pushed on Mario's right shoulder.

There was little automobile traffic, although they dodged assorted hazards such as wandering dogs and children playing ball in the street. They slowly made their way out to a quiet country road lined with corn and hayfields.

Mario turned around and said to his brother. "What do you see, Charlie? Anything interesting?"

Charlie opened his mouth to respond but was interrupted by the shrill call of a woman gardening in her yard by the road.

"Young man! I suggest that you keep your eyes on the road!"

As the car passed by, Charlie replied, "Oh, he doesn't need to watch the road." Mario drove on with a big grin on his face, leaving a very puzzled woman behind.

• •

GEOGRAPHY LESSON

"MARIO, YOU MAY join Jane at the map table," said sixth-grade teacher Miss Campton in her crisp, no-nonsense voice. "You are to feel each state, read the name, and put it back in the proper place."

Thirteen-year-old Mario's heart leapt with joy. He couldn't believe his good fortune. This was his first opportunity to speak to Jane, and even more fortuitous, he could show her his knowledge of the state of Indiana. He'd been interested in geography since he was old enough to learn the names of streets in his neighborhood. On his trip to Italy at age five, he'd surprised his mother by memorizing every town that the train would pass through on its way from Muncie to New York City. Longitude and latitude were fascinating concepts to him, and he learned where the major cities were located according to those numbers. Even though he was too young to leave the school unescorted, he learned the names and patterns of the Indianapolis streets. He wanted to know all he could about his environment, as someday he'd need to know how to go somewhere on his own. Street signs would be of no use to him.

The map table was where the teacher kept a specially designed map of the United States. Like a puzzle, each piece was the outline of a state. Students were to take out a state, identify it by shape, and put it back in the proper spot. Each state was labeled in Braille, with raised outlines indicating rivers. Mounds indicated hills, and mountains were mounds with sharper points.

Jane was relieved when she heard the teacher call Mario up to the table. She liked the quiet, studious boy. His precise and intelligent answers to the teacher's questions were unlike any of the other boys'. He didn't make vulgar sounds or frighten her like the other boys.

"Mario," Jane whispered. "I'm terrible at geography. I don't know how to do these maps."

From the moment he first heard Jane's voice in the fourth grade, Mario was smitten. He had no idea what she looked like, but it didn't matter. He liked what he heard—the softness of her voice and her intelligent answers to the teacher's questions. Her voice sounded kind, never sharp. He longed to hear more, but boys were forbidden to speak to the girls outside of class. In the mid-1920s, the school had separate dining halls, playgrounds, and indoor playrooms for the sexes. Between classes, hall monitors made sure that nothing was said, nor physical contact made between boys and girls. Only in sixth grade did the school begin to allow limited interactions between the sexes during instructional time.

"It's not so hard. Look! Feel this one. It's the state of Florida!" He held the cutout of the state and reached towards Jane. The thirteen-year-old extended her hand. Not wanting to drop it, Mario covered her soft hand with his own as he passed the piece to her. The electricity startled them both, and Mario quickly removed his hand. It was the first time he'd ever touched a girl's hand. He had no sisters and only played with Charlie and their male neighborhood friends. Jane also had no experience with the opposite sex. Since she had no brothers, and the school rules strictly prohibited any touching between the sexes, she'd never felt the roughness of a boy's hand. Both Mario and Jane liked that new sensation but remembered to keep focused on their assignment.

Jane held the puzzle piece with her left hand and ran her fingers around the smooth edges. "I didn't know that Florida was so long and skinny! Where's Indiana? I've always wondered how our state is shaped."

Encouraged to show off his knowledge, Mario thought it proper to take her hand and show her the state. With his hand over hers, they traced the major Indiana rivers and felt the southern Indiana hills. The teacher was apparently not concerned with enforcing the "no touching" rule, and allowed the two to continue exploring the puzzle.

With Mario's help, Jane began to understand the geography of the state. While she'd seen maps many times in public school, she'd only been able to see splotches of color, such as blue for the Great Lakes. But she couldn't see the outlines on regular maps, so she had no idea of the shape of each state.

Mario and Jane spent a long time that day feeling the shape of each state and putting them back into the correct place. Both were surprised that the teacher had allowed them so much time together. But neither complained. And neither forgot that day at school.

• :

PROHIBITION PROFITS

IN 1920, CONGRESS passed the Eighteenth Amendment to the United States Constitution, outlawing the production and sale of liquor. Alcohol was blamed for family violence, alcoholism, and political corruption; it was thought that those ills would be solved by Prohibition. Making alcohol illegal, however, did not stop people from drinking. Men bought bootleg liquor and often drove to deserted country roads to drink it, tossing the empty glass bottles into roadside ditches.

Eleven-year-old Charlie saw their littering as an investment opportunity. He picked up discarded medicine, milk, and Coke bottles, took them home, and washed them. He then sold them to the men he knew from the sidewalk outside of his father's store. Antonio apparently either didn't mind the men's presence or was too frightened to ask them to leave. It's possible that they were "protecting" his store for a fee. In any case, the bootleggers were glad to have the clean bottles and paid Charlie ten cents each—a huge sum for the times, equivalent to $1.29 in today's dollars.

Soon, Charlie learned that he could get fifteen cents a bottle if the cap was clean and not rusty. Most bottles that he found had no caps, as they were discarded in the rush to open the bottle. Since caps were hard to find, Charlie went to a wholesale drug supply company and purchased a gross of caps. He quickly sold out and repeated the process, greatly increasing his profits.

Along with his thriving bottle business, Charlie worked at his father's store. Antonio paid his son $10 a week to work from 8:00 p.m. until midnight. They sold popcorn to patrons of nearby movie theaters (at that time, no snacks were sold at the theater). Antonio also sold fudge, tobacco, chewing tobacco, sodas, malts, milkshakes, and warm roasted nuts. For those customers who were constipated, they had prune juice available. If someone had a headache and indigestion, Alka- Seltzer was offered.

By the time that he'd graduated from high school, Charlie had saved over $1,000. He wanted to use the money to go back to the family's village in Italy, San Pietro in Campo. With Charlie paying his own expenses, Antonio and Eletta decided that they could afford to take Mario and go back for a visit.

While their parents visited with their Italian kinfolk, Charlie and Mario were free to travel around Italy unsupervised. They used train passes to take day trips to wherever looked interesting. Each day brought a different adventure, sometimes hiking in the Dolomite Mountains or exploring Lucca and other nearby Tuscan towns.

Their grandmother's village was located near the Apuan Alps in Tuscany. Charlie and Mario often took daylong hikes, developing a system where Charlie led and Mario followed, holding Charlie's left hand with his right. Mario could follow exactly behind him and even learned to step over rocks without Charlie warning him. He followed his brother's movements; while stepping over rocks, Charlie moved differently than simply walking. Mario felt the difference and imitated his brother, rarely tripping.

One morning, they decided to climb to the top of a nearby mountain. It was not an easy climb, and they had no equipment. The narrow trail went between two peaks at 4,000 feet; the wind blew hard at right angles, forcing the hikers to lean into the wind and causing them to be unbalanced.

"Mario, there's a little path here," Charlie yelled into his ear. "We're going from one peak to the next. You walk behind me. Hold on to my belt. And no matter what, don't let go. Don't step on either side, or else you'll go down, down, down."

Mario did what he was told, and slowly, they made their way along the dangerous path. Fighting the wind and hoping that it wouldn't knock him over, Mario couldn't hear any further instructions from Charlie, only the roar of the wind. Occasionally, he heard the tinkling of sheep bells off in the distance. He couldn't tell where the flocks were—they could have been up in the sky or way down on the Earth—as sound carried great distances in the mountains. But the bells were a nice distraction from the fear that if he took a misstep, he'd fall down the rocky mountainside and take his adored brother with him.

Complicating the difficult passage was the damp grass, which made the path extremely slippery. There was nothing but his brother to hold on to, no barrier to stop a long slide to a terrifying death. Mario's heart was racing as they finally made it to the other side. His hand was cramped from holding Charlie's belt so tightly.

"Charlie, let's rest for a minute." His hands were shaking as he gasped for air.

"Here's a big rock. You can sit down here while we catch our breath," said Charlie as he took Mario's hand and put it on the rock so that his brother would know the location and height of the boulder.

Mario nodded, felt the top of the rock for smoothness, and sat down, avoiding the jagged far edge.

Charlie continued, "I was scared, too. Good thing that you stayed right behind me, Mario. You could have fallen a very long way down the mountain. I wish that you could see this view. I can see little white dots of sheep way down there. And there's a village. I can see the church steeple from here."

"Maybe I'm glad that I couldn't see how high up we were. You were a good guide, Charlie, but let's not do that again. That wind was really blowing, and I could barely hear you. Promise me that we'll go a different way home!"

* * *

Later that summer, the eighteen- and fifteen-year-old boys received permission to take overnight trips alone. Their first destination was Venice, where they spent hours exploring and enjoying the bustle of the city.

"Charlie let's go for a gondola ride. I'm tired of walking," complained Mario.

"It's early in our trip. We should save our money," Charlie replied. "But it does look like fun. Let's walk over the bridge. I think that there's one on the other side."

Mario smiled in anticipation. He'd heard the water softly lapping against the side of the canal whenever a boat would pass. And many of the oarsmen had beautiful voices, singing as they poled their ways down the narrow canals. Sitting in a gondola, smelling the fresh air off the ocean, and moving without having to walk on his sore feet—Mario couldn't think of a better way to spend a warm afternoon in Venice.

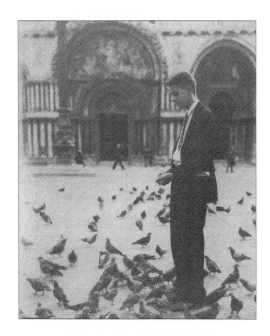

Mario in St. Mark's Square, Venice

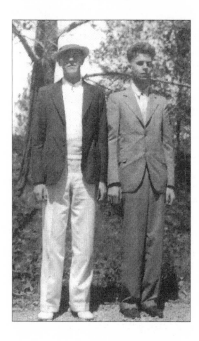

Charles and Mario Pieroni, ages 18 and 15

Leaving Venice the next day, they took the train to the nearby city of Trieste, located across the Adriatic Sea from Venice. That evening, they enjoyed a few Serbian beers in a large, open piazza and were walking back to their hotel when Mario heard a very odd whistle coming from the nearby wharves.

"You know, Charlie, that's a funny sounding whistle. I wonder what type of boat that is," said Mario.

"Well, let's go see!"

With Mario holding Charlie's elbow, the boys ran down the narrow cobblestone street, their heavy footsteps echoing off the dark buildings. Mario heard the whistle blow again and said, "There! It's coming from the right. We're close!"

The boys rounded a corner and slowed to a fast walk. Mario felt the warm sea breeze on his face and deeply inhaled the ocean scent of fish and brine. He clicked his tongue, which he often did to determine how high a ceiling was or where a wall ended. There was no echo from nearby buildings. "Aren't we at the docks? It feels very open here."

The whistle sounded again, this time so loudly that both boys covered their ears. "It's a ferry," said Charlie.

"Let's find out where it goes," replied Mario.

Charlie asked a worker and found that it was going to Izola. They'd never heard of Izola. "Sir, where is Izola?"

"It's just across the bay. The boat is ready to leave. Are you coming now or not?" asked the worker.

The brothers looked at each other and together said, "We're coming."

They boarded the ferry and discovered that they were the only passengers. A bored crew member was happy to have somebody to talk with, and noting their American accents, asked the boys in Italian where they were from. They conversed during the half-hour ride, happily telling him about their travels around Italy.

Approaching the end of the trip, Mario asked, "Sir, what time does the ferry go back to Trieste?" thinking that it was time to go back to the hotel for some sleep.

"There is no service back to Trieste until morning," he replied.

"What? Well, gosh!" said Mario. "We don't know Izola. We've never even heard of it. We need a place to sleep."

"Well, you can just stay on the ferry all night, if you want to. You can sleep on any of these benches."

When the ferry arrived in port, the crew closed down the boat and left the boys alone. It became very quiet. Luckily, it was a warm summer night, and there was no rain. The wooden benches were hard, but they managed to get some sleep. The next morning, the ferry returned them back to Trieste, where they boarded a train to Postumia, in what is now Slovenia, but at the time was part of Italy.

Charlie had seen many posters advertising a symphony concert to be held deep below ground in the caverns of Postumia, and Mario couldn't wait to go. He wanted to experience both the cave and hear the concert led by a famous conductor. What would music sound like in the bowels of the Earth? He expected the acoustics to be amazing and much different from those in a typical concert hall.

The only way to reach the concert was by a small, open-air train car that went down about two miles into the cave. With Mario's left hand tightly holding on to the arm of his seat, and his right arm entwined with Charlie's, Mario leaned forward and enjoyed feeling the car's motion as it rolled farther into the cool earth. He smiled as he clicked his tongue often, gauging the size of the tunnel.

"Brrr! It's cold in here, Charlie. I wish that I had my jacket. And the ceiling sounds pretty low. Do I need to duck?" asked Mario.

"You don't need to duck, but you're right. The ceiling is about three feet above our heads. I can't see much. It's real dark down here. They have lanterns every so often. I guess there's just not much to see yet."

The train arrived at the opening of a large cavern filled with thousands of people waiting for the orchestra to begin. Mario was not disappointed. The music echoed off the cave walls, creating a magical effect. He was thrilled with the once-in-a-lifetime experience.

After the concert, the boys toured the cave, with Charlie describing the otherworldly formations rising from below and hanging from the ceiling. He guided Mario to a particularly large one close to the path and said, "Mario, here's a stalactite." He took his brother's hand and gently put it on the wet rock. "Look how big it is, and it's hanging down from the ceiling!"

Mario explored the rough surfaces with both hands. "This thing is huge. And it feels very rough. I didn't know that a stalactite would have such a strange shape." Over his lifetime he would visit many caves, during which he learned that his touch damaged the delicate structures. While disappointed that he could no longer touch stalagmites and stalactites to understand their shapes, he still enjoyed the descriptions provided by companions and the cool, echoing atmosphere. The music from the concert of 1929 reverberated frequently in his mind; reliving that day and recounting the story brought him much pleasure during his life.

In August, the family traveled by train to Rome to sightsee and enjoy Mario's favorite opera, *Rigoletto*. Late on the afternoon of the performance, Charlie asked Mario to go for a walk before leaving for the opera. Mario reluctantly agreed to a short excursion, insisting on returning soon enough so that they wouldn't be late for the opening curtain. The teens set off from their hotel and walked about fifteen minutes when Charlie suddenly stopped.

"Mario, we're lost. I don't know where we are or how to get back to the hotel."

"Aren't we close to the Victor Emmanuel Monument?" asked Mario. "There are so many people here that we must be close to something important."

"Let's go down this alley. I just want to get out of this crowd," said Charlie. Once out of the crush of people, he took out his map and held the large piece of paper up against the building, trying to figure out the way back.

Suddenly, Mario heard heavy footsteps coming toward them. Loud voices spoke rapid Italian, so fast that neither boy understood.

"Mario, they're soldiers!" Charlie whispered as their arms were grabbed and held behind their backs.

"What are you doing?" asked one of the men.

"We're just trying to figure out where we are," replied Charlie in Italian.

"You must come with us."

"But we didn't do anything wrong!"

"You must come with us to the station. Now!"

Italy was a police state under Mussolini, and the boys were terrified that they would be arrested.

Mario protested, telling them that they had to go to an opera and were American citizens. He pulled out his passport and showed them, thinking that it would protect him, and they would let them go.

"We don't care who you are or about your passport. You must come with us."

At the police station, they were questioned for about an hour. They had been loitering next to Mussolini's headquarters, which had attracted the soldiers' attention. Charlie had picked the wrong spot to look at a map. Finally, the soldiers decided that the boys were harmless and released them. Shaken, the boys ran back to the hotel, arriving just in time to attend the opera with their parents.

* * *

Italy was not the only country where the brothers had adventures. In the summer of 1933, Mario was nineteen and about to enter his senior year at the School for the Blind. Charles (as he was known by then) and two of his college friends, George Dyke and James Smith, decided to take a road trip to Montreal, Canada. When Charles invited Mario to come along, Mario enthusiastically agreed. They would take Charles' newly purchased car, a used Chrysler 77 coupe, complete with a rumble seat in back. America was still in Prohibition, but Canada was wet. The thirsty friends thought that a trip to Canada would be the perfect way to vacation and celebrate summer with legal beer.

The four young men began the journey at midnight shortly after Charles closed the confectionery. Tired from a long day selling candy and tobacco, Charles asked James to drive. George and Charles settled onto the front leather bench seat, while Mario climbed into the rumble seat. He stretched out sideways to accommodate his long legs and enjoyed the cool night breeze caressing his face. It didn't take long for Mario to discover why it was called the "rumble seat." The combined noise of the wind, engine, and tires made it impossible for Mario to hear his companions' conversation, but he was too sleepy to care. He drifted off to sleep as the old car sped through the night.

The trip went smoothly until shortly after 2:00 a.m., when on a two-lane road, their car sideswiped another going the opposite direction. The loud bang woke everyone up, including the driver. They stopped and discovered that the rope holding a metal oilcan to the running board had been torn off, but fortunately, there was no damage to the car. The other car didn't stop, so the boys assumed that it had no damage. It was a close call; the group decided it was as much their driver's fault as the other guy's, so they put James on "probation" and switched drivers.

They continued through Ohio and crossed into Canada at Buffalo, New York. By then, James was back at the wheel. It was midafternoon, with good visibility, but James was driving too fast when he came over a hill and saw the back of an old man driving a white horse and wagon. He couldn't stop in time, and the coupe bumped the wagon's rear.

Charles hopped out of the car while the man inspected his property. The French-Canadian furiously spoke French and made it clear that they were at fault. Charles spoke to him in a soothing voice, and finally the man began to calm down. Charles offered him $3.00 for whatever he claimed was wrong with his wagon. He took the money and they drove away. That was James' last time behind the wheel.

The group stayed in Montreal for two days, sightseeing and relaxing in bars. The car had been parked in a parking garage across from their hotel. The next morning, when Charles tried to start the car for the trip home, they found that the choke wire had been cut.

A vandal had cut a piece out of it. Mario theorized that someone wanted to make some business for a local garage, but the boys didn't know why their car had been singled out. Frightened that someone wanted to harm them, they found a mechanic who fixed it for a good price and made a hasty exit from Montreal.

As they were approaching the U.S. border, George reminded them that it was still Prohibition in the U.S. and that they should at least stop and get one last good bottle of beer. They pulled into a small grocery, where they purchased a large jug of Black Horse Beer. As they drove south toward the border, it occurred to them that they couldn't bring the beer into the country. They turned off the highway and drove down a little country road. There was no traffic, and no houses were in sight, so they stopped to drink the beer. It was warm, and tasted awful, but they drank it anyway just because they couldn't once they crossed the border.

Mario decided that he'd like to drive in Canada and insisted on getting behind the wheel. Charles reluctantly agreed and climbed into the rumble seat, where he stood leaning forward so that he could reach Mario's shoulders. Mario drove slowly but steadily on the narrow gravel road. Luckily, there were no other cars.

"We're coming up to a little bridge, Mario. Just stay straight and hold tight when we hit the edge. You'll feel a bump," said Charles.

"Okay," Mario answered and tightened his grip on the vibrating steering wheel. The rubber tires bounced onto the wood planks. Mario felt pressure on his right shoulder, so he angled the car to the right. Immediately he heard a loud cracking noise and felt the car sideswipe the protective wood railing. He jerked the wheel left as the railing fell into the creek, and jammed on the brakes as Charles yelled, "Why didn't you do what I told you? You almost ran us off the bridge!"

"You pushed my right shoulder!"

"No, I didn't. I told you to go left!"

The brothers had a loud discussion, with Charles insisting that he had pushed Mario's left shoulder, and that he should have edged left instead of going right. Realizing that he couldn't win the argument with his brother, Mario sighed and climbed back into the rumble seat so Charles could get them off the bridge.

That argument was never resolved. Over seventy years later, at Mario's ninetieth birthday party, Charles told his version of the story. Mario claimed that Charles was still wrong, but they agreed to blame the Black Horse Beer.

• ••

HIGH SCHOOL ROMANCE

JANE'S SUMMER OF 1929 was not nearly as exciting as Mario's adventures in Italy. She was home on the farm, but although she was fifteen years old, her mother refused to allow her to do any chores or help in the kitchen. Bessie didn't know how to teach her daughter life skills; Jane was more trouble to have around than helpful. Jane was frustrated that her mother wouldn't help her learn to cook or sew and looked forward to learning those skills at school. At least the teachers believed she could learn to do things that sighted people could do. She was disheartened that her mother, who'd vowed to make her the happiest baby in the county, was now making her unhappy by telling her all the things that she couldn't do.

Time at home seemed endless; the routine varied little. Jane was lonely on the farm and missed her school friends, especially Mario. She wondered what he was doing and imagined that he was probably having fun in Muncie with his brother. She eagerly looked forward to September when she could see Mario again and hear about his summer.

When Jane arrived back at school, she learned that Mario was in Italy and would not return until after Thanksgiving. She was deeply disappointed that he'd be gone for months, but school without Mario was still better than sitting at home on the isolated farm. Classwork, friends, and activities helped to fill the void.

At last, Mario returned to school in December. Jane perked up when she heard his voice again in English class and was anxious to hear about his travels. As the smartest students in the class, it didn't take them long to finish their work assignments. Since they had extra time, the kind teacher broke school rules and allowed them to talk quietly in the back of the classroom. Mario told Jane about his trip to Italy, enthusiastically giving many details about life on board the ship, the noises it made, and the passengers he'd met. He and Charles had gone hiking in the mountains, explored villages and cities, and been detained by some of Mussolini's police in Rome. Jane listened raptly, hardly believing that Mario's parents had allowed him, at age fifteen, to roam Italy with just his brother.

* * *

Jane finished brushing her short, wavy brown hair and carefully set the brush down in its place on top of her dresser. The fifteen-year-old eighth grader wanted everything to be perfect, even though her date wouldn't be able to see her at the Valentine's Day dance.

"How do I look, Margaret?" Jane asked her roommate as she twirled in her pink, pleated dress that her mother had made especially for her.

Margaret, who had some vision, said, "Jane, your dress looks perfect on you. I love your lace collar. May I touch your collar? I love the feel of lace."

"Sure, you can feel it," Jane answered as she leaned forward for her friend.

"Oh, it feels soft. And if I look very closely, I can see the lace flowers. They're very pretty." Margaret's head was only about five inches away from Jane's collar. Feeling uncomfortably close, Jane stepped back. She was still traumatized by the memory of her first day at the school when the girls' hands touched her all over to see what she looked like. "Well, it's time for us to leave for the Athletic Club. I can't wait to see Mario. It's our first real date!"

"Don't you just hate how they will only let us talk to boys at these dances? We only have three dances a year—Halloween, Christmas, and Valentine's Day. That's not enough time to spend with the boys," said Margaret.

"I know. We're already fifteen years old and almost grown up. We should be allowed to talk to the boys, but the school has their silly rules. Come on, let's go!"

The Indianapolis Athletic Club provided a luxurious setting in downtown just a few blocks away from the school. The ballroom had dark wood paneling, with crystal chandeliers lighting the expansive space. The many oil paintings lining the walls were lost on the students. Those with limited vision were too excited to spend time appreciating art.

Mario sat on an overstuffed armchair near the ballroom's entrance anxiously waiting to hear the sound of Jane's voice. He rubbed his sweaty palms on his best suit pants and tried to swallow, though his dry mouth felt like cotton. He hoped that Jane would arrive soon so that he could offer her a trip to the punch bowl. It would be a good conversation starter and help to quench his thirst. As much as he wanted to waltz with her, he'd never danced before and worried about stepping on her feet.

"Mario! Jane's here," said Henry, his partially sighted roommate. "Come on, I'll walk with you to meet her."

"Thanks," said Mario as he quickly rose from his chair and took his friend's elbow. "Hold on tight, Mario. I know that you're in a hurry to see Jane," Henry said while quickly threading their way through the crowd. Moments later, he exclaimed, "Here she is! Jane, this is Mario."

Mario felt his heart beat faster. "Hello, Jane. How are you? Would you like some punch?"

"Hello, Mario. Yes, sure, I'd like some punch."

"May I have your hand? Henry will show us where the refreshments are," Mario asked as he reached out, hoping that she would accept.

"Oh yes, this is a big room, and I don't want to lose you."

Mario smiled as he gently but firmly took her hand, hoping that his palms weren't too sweaty. The touch of her hand electrified him, and though he couldn't see her face, he was certain that she felt the same way. This was going to be a wonderful night.

When a talented student, Howard Bloom, began playing waltzes on the grand piano, Mario took Jane into his arms for the first time. What a feeling! With his hand on her back, he realized that he'd never touched a girl's dress before. The fabric was soft, yet crisply ironed, and he felt it move as Jane swayed in time to the music. He didn't dare dance too closely; the superintendent and teachers were everywhere, watching for any improprieties. It didn't matter that neither knew how to dance. Everyone shuffled from side to side; Mario wasn't worried about bumping into other couples. He could hear if they got too close; and since many students still had some vision, they were able to avoid collisions.

Jane was surprised at how tall Mario was; she reached her left hand up higher than she'd expected to on his shoulder. She was aware of his long fingers clasped around her right hand, holding her firmly yet gently. He smelled of Lifebuoy soap; that was a good sign, since so many of the boys didn't seem to care about personal hygiene, and she'd scrunched her nose up in disgust when passing them by in the hall.

Mario was different from the other boys in the school. He was gentlemanly and intelligent, with good manners. The conversation flowed easily between them, making each wanting to learn more about the other. His smooth, cultured voice captivated her, and Mario memorized everything that Jane said. He wanted to relive every detail of that marvelous night; those thoughts would keep him company during the long periods when he couldn't be with her.

Time passed quickly, and all too soon, fellow student Howard Bloom stopped playing the piano. The superintendent picked up the microphone and announced, "The dance is over. Please release your partners. I hope that you had a good time, but now it's time for the girls to head to their bus. The boys will follow in a few minutes. Remember that boys and girls may not talk to each other in the halls, dining room, or classrooms. Good night."

Mario turned to Jane and said, "Thank you for dancing with me. I really liked chatting with you, and I'll miss talking with you at school."

"I know, I hate that we can't talk to each other there. I wish that the dance wasn't over."

"Jane, it's time to go," said a chaperone. "I'll walk with you back to the bus."

Mario reluctantly released Jane's hand, but not before squeezing it gently. He wanted her to know by his touch just how much he liked her. He'd savored every moment of the evening.

Mario would not forget that night.

* * *

Jane and Mario's eighth grade year, 1929–1930, was significant for the school itself. The city of Indianapolis had decided in 1920 to build a War Memorial Plaza to honor all Indiana veterans, and the school, originally built in 1850, was located on property needed for the new memorial. The city decided to move the school to a sixty-three–acre site about six miles north of downtown. Construction of the new campus began in 1926 , building dorms, classrooms, administration, and support buildings. When Jane and Mario finished eighth grade in 1930, the old school was shuttered and demolished.

Jane and Mario were eager to explore the new campus when they arrived in September 1930. As sixteen-year-old freshmen, they were still kept apart by the strict rules, so they discovered their new environment with friends. While the girls were closely supervised and not allowed to go by themselves, Mario and his friends roamed the acres of hills, forests, and grassy areas unchaperoned. He appreciated the peaceful quiet of the neighborhood and listened avidly to birdsongs.

Occasionally, a train rumbled by on tracks behind the campus, interrupting the birds, but Mario didn't mind. He loved the sound of passenger and freight cars clicking by and dreamed of one day taking the train to distant exotic locations. For more immediate adventures, the boys would walk to the school's entrance and take the streetcar or bus to explore the city or shop downtown. They didn't have much money, but they enjoyed exploring the growing city and learning their way around.

* * *

Open only to residents of Indiana, the School for the Blind was free and taught children of varying abilities. Some, like Jane and Mario, were totally blind. Others had some vision but not enough to function in regular school. Even more varied were the intellectual capacities of the students. Some were of average intelligence, while others were far below. A few were gifted musically, while others used their hands to make crafts. Mario wasn't interested in learning chair caning or other trades. Those trades would not allow him to earn enough to marry Jane and raise a family. He was determined to get an education and become financially independent of his parents.

Taught by sighted teachers, the curriculum was divided into three sections: Literary, Music, and Industrial Departments. The Literary Department offered classes in mathematics, English, social studies, science, and typing on print and Braille typewriters. The Music Department admitted all students to the chorus; if a child showed musical promise, he was given piano, violin, or organ lessons. Students without musical talent nor academically inclined, were enrolled in the Industrial Department. Boys were offered classes in piano tuning, mop and broom making, and chair caning. Girls learned sewing, knitting, and basket making.

Mario and Jane were members of the Literary Department throughout high school and took the more advanced classes. Both enjoyed English, reading classic books, and learning to write research papers.

Mario enjoyed plane geometry. The teacher drew diagrams to make raised lines that were perceptible to the touch. Angles were marked by Braille letters. Remarkably, he learned to use a compass and straight edge to draw his own geometrical proofs.

Jane's favorite subject was English, and she especially enjoyed books that detailed how people lived in foreign countries. She devoured *Jane Eyre*, relishing the romance, relationships, and drama.

Having grown up on a central Indiana farm and living in an institution, Jane often felt isolated and lonely. Books enabled her to escape to faraway places and to meet more interesting people than she ever could on her own.

As Jane's family did not yet have a telephone, the only way to communicate with her family was to write letters. Jane often wrote in Braille to her sister Irma and mother. Self-taught, both were able to read and write Braille, although Bessie was more proficient. Jane's sister Ruth wasn't interested in learning Braille. She depended upon Bessie to read Jane's letters to her. When Ruth wrote back, Jane needed to find a classmate with enough vision to read Ruth's letters to her.

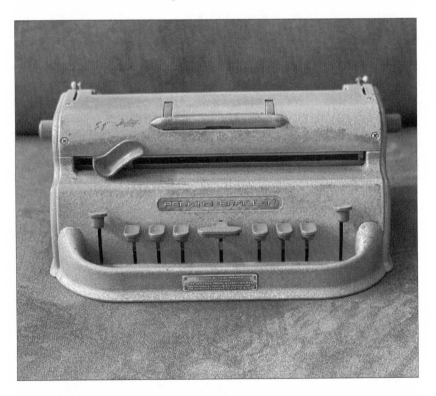

Mario's Perkins Braille Typewriter

Jane had longed to write more private letters to her sisters, letters that her mother didn't have to read or translate. In high school, Jane took typing classes for a print typewriter, while Mario took typing classes on both print and Braille typewriters. Jane could take notes in Braille with a slate and stylus; she didn't feel the need to learn the Braille typewriter.

Typing class wasn't easy, but they relished another opportunity for independence. It took a lot of practice memorizing where each letter was located on the keyboard, but at last, they could write on regular paper, and a sighted person could read it! Jane began a lifetime of writing letters on a typewriter, including those she would write to her children many years later.

Although not taught as a skill to earn money, Mario's ability to type on both the Braille and print typewriters would prove to be much more useful in making a living than making and selling brooms. In addition to his typing skills, Mario would use his memory, words, and communication skills to make more money than he could dream of while in school.

• ••
•

DARING COURTSHIP

BEGINNING IN HIGH school, the sexes were allowed to join coed enrichment activities such as the choir, orchestra, and the Philomathean Society, which sponsored plays and the annual spring operetta. Although it was quite prestigious to have a leading role in the operetta, Jane and Mario had no desire to spend rehearsal evenings out on stage trying to remember their lines.

Instead, they joined the chorus. There was a lot of time that the chorus had nothing to do; the boys were supposed to be in the boys' anteroom and the girls in theirs on the opposite side of the stage. Knowing that Jane was so close by frustrated Mario. He figured out that Jane and he could get behind the thick curtain on either side of the stage and walk slowly until they met in the middle. They could speak softly, and more importantly, talk privately. They even held hands, which was quite daring. If caught, they would have been reported to the school superintendent, who in turn would have told their parents. But they were never discovered.

As the date of the performance drew near, Mario was saddened at the thought of less time with Jane. He thought that there had to be another way for them to communicate. The teachers and governesses who provided custodial care closely monitored the students for evidence of forbidden communications, ostensibly to prevent any opportunities for romantic rendezvous. If caught, the missives would be read and parents notified, which would be extremely embarrassing.

During a break at the last rehearsal before Thanksgiving of their junior year, when Mario and Jane were already nineteen years old, Mario held Jane's hand as they huddled behind the theatre's curtain.

"Jane, don't you send your laundry home?" he whispered.

"Yes," she replied. "I put it in a cloth bag, and the school ships it to Mom. Why do you ask?"

"Because I can send a Braille letter to your home address, and when your mom gets it, she could hold the letter until she finishes washing your clothes. Then she could hide the letter in with all your laundry. When you get your clean clothes, you'll also get my letter!"

"Ohhh, I see. And it takes my mom a long time to read Braille, so I don't think that she'd bother to read your letters. But how will I write back to you?"

"Easy. I have it all figured out. You write to me in Braille. Address the envelope to me on a print typewriter and put the letter in with your dirty clothes. Then when your mother finds it, she mails it in another envelope to my mom. Then Mom will send it to me," explained Mario. "My Mom can't read Braille, so we don't have to worry about her."

"But what if my Mom won't do it? Maybe she'll say no and get us in trouble."

"I think that she'll do anything for you. She feels terrible that you're blind and have to be here. Just ask her, please?"

"What about your Mom, Mario? Would she really help us?"

"She'll do it. Just like your Mom, mine has always felt terrible about my blindness. Let's try it. Won't it be fun to get letters and fool the governesses? Besides, we're both good at typing in Braille and with a print typewriter. We can address our own letters with no problem."

At Thanksgiving that year, Jane asked Bessie, and Mario recruited Eletta to help in carrying out their scheme. Much to their relief, both mothers readily agreed, and almost two years of clandestine letter writing began.

When summer vacation arrived, they continued corresponding, albeit directly and without maternal help. Summers were especially lonely for Jane; waiting for the arrival of the rural mail carrier's automobile gave her something to look forward to each day. Hearing his car chugging down the road, Jane's face lit up in anticipation. Perhaps she would have a letter from Mario! On the special days when a letter was delivered, she was delighted to open the fat envelope of heavy Braille paper with the raised dots. She happily settled down in her favorite chair to read and re-read Mario's news.

Since Jane's family didn't have a telephone, letters were the only way for the couple to communicate. Muncie was only about sixty miles away from the farm near Wabash, but without transportation, the distance felt like six hundred miles.

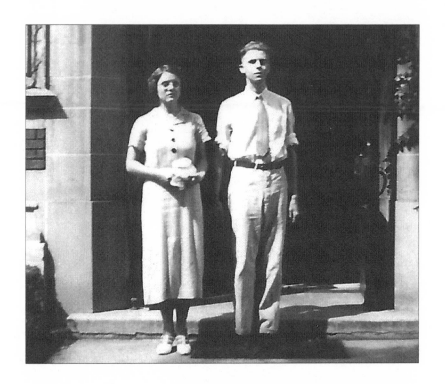

Jane Small, Mario Pieroni
Indiana School for the Blind

$$\bullet \ \ \bullet \ \bullet$$

SWEPT AWAY

DURING THE GREAT Depression of the early 1930s, vocations were very limited for blind men. Some were musicians, a few sold candy at county courthouses, and others were reduced to begging on a street corner. Mario wanted nothing to do with those options. He couldn't earn a living to support himself, much less a wife and family.

Since it was hard for anyone to earn a living during the Depression, much less a blind man, the school taught all middle and high school boys broom making and chair caning skills in the hopes that they would learn a viable trade. Caned-bottom chairs were common, and the weaving was easily broken. Teachers hoped to inspire the students, telling them about recent graduates who worked as chair repairmen. One lucky alumnus, whose family had a little money, bought some simple machinery and set up a broom making workshop in the family's garage. After making several brooms, the young man peddled them door-to-door. Though he couldn't earn enough to support himself, he at least had the dignity of earning spending money.

When Mario and his close friend, Arthur, heard that story, they wondered if they could sell brooms, too. They convinced school officials to allow them to purchase the brooms they made for ten cents and sell them for thirty cents. They were allowed to keep the profits, which provided a strong incentive. It was also a good excuse to leave the campus on weekends and gain valuable experience traveling without the assistance of a sighted person.

On a breezy April afternoon, nineteen-year-old Mario and Arthur boarded the streetcar at the stop by the entrance to the School for the Blind. The driver, who knew many of the students who rode his route, greeted them with a friendly "Hello, boys! What are you going to do with all those brooms?"

"Sell 'em, sir!" Mario replied.

"Well, good for you. Do you have a destination in mind?"

"Yes, sir. Our teacher said to try Elm Street," said Arthur.

"All right, I'll let you know when we get to Elm Street."

Fifteen minutes later the steel streetcar wheels screeched to a halt. The driver opened the folding door and said, "Boys, this is the corner of Elm and Mulberry streets. It's a nice neighborhood. You should be able to make some sales today."

"Thank you, sir," they replied in unison as they climbed down the steps and emerged into the warm spring sun. The streetcar's brakes released with a loud whoosh of air, and the driver rang the bell as a friendly farewell.

Mario and Arthur, also totally blind, paused at the corner to get their bearings. "The driver said that this is the corner of Elm and Mulberry streets. I'll take this side of Elm and you take the other. We'll meet at the next corner," said Mario.

"That's fine with me," replied Arthur. "Good luck. I'll see you soon." The boys shouldered the brooms they'd made earlier that week at the school's workshop and began walking, hoping to make some sales at the houses lining the block.

Swishing his cane back and forth, Mario walked down the sidewalk, clicking his tongue against the roof of his mouth, and listening for the sound to bounce back. Based on that sound's characteristics, he was able to tell if an object was a tree or something bigger, such as a house.

Homes were built close to the sidewalk. Many had porches equipped with swings so the owners could enjoy fresh air and watch the neighborhood goings-on. They were built on narrow lots, often only ten feet apart. The high density made it easier for the boys to locate the front doors and provided more opportunities for making a sale.

With his brooms standing upright, his left hand holding them steady, Mario knocked on the wooden door and stood back as he waited for someone to answer. A nearby bird sang its cheerful song, which Mario, who knew most bird calls, immediately identified as a cardinal. Mario smiled to himself. Cardinals were good luck, and he hoped that its appearance would mean a sale.

Dressed in his Sunday suit and tie, Mario stood straighter when he heard the door open. "Yes, what do you want?" asked an older woman's voice.

"Hello, ma'am. My name is Mario, and I'm a student at the School for the Blind. I made these brooms just this week and thought that you would appreciate the superb quality of the materials and workmanship."

"Let me see one."

Mario held one out for her to examine. He was happy that he got this far. Many times, the person said no and slammed the door in his face. He smiled at her and said, "You can never have too many brooms. And I know that you like to keep a very clean house."

The woman hesitated. "I don't know. But it is a nice broom."

Mario tried to close the sale. "This one will last longer than the kind you find in a general store. And it's only thirty cents!"

"Thirty cents is a lot of money. But you seem like a nice boy, and you did a good job on it. Just a minute. I'll bring you three dimes."

"Thank you, ma'am. I really do appreciate it."

Mario was delighted to have made the sale. He now had a little spending money and one less broom to lug around.

He continued down the block, selling two more brooms. Arriving at the corner, Mario stood and turned his head to bask in the sun. The warmth on his face relaxed him as he listened to the birds sing their spring mating songs. Mario also listened for Arthur's voice calling out his name.

Tired of waiting, and wondering where his friend was, Mario decided to cross the street and go back to meet him. He hesitated before stepping off the curb, listening for the loud rumbling noise of approaching automobiles. Hearing nothing but birdsong, Mario stepped down onto the street and soon felt the road begin to rise. Brick streets were built with a higher center, allowing rainwater to drain into sewers. He knew that he was halfway across when he felt the bricks start going down toward the curb.

Mario reached the other side and turned down the sidewalk, calling his friend's name.

"Arthur? Where are you?"

Receiving no answer, he continued down the sidewalk, calling out every few feet. Mario was puzzled and began to worry. Arthur should have been at the corner by now. He knew not to ever enter someone's house, and he should have been able to hear his name. How could he be lost in just one block?

Mario called even louder, "Arthur, where *are* you?"

This time, a faint voice responded. Mario turned his head in the direction of the voice and yelled, "Hey! I hear you. But you sound so far away!"

"I'm down here! I'm down in somebody's cellar."

Mario began walking toward his friend's voice. "I'm coming! Keep talking to me so I can find you."

"I got up on the porch and instead of finding the door, I fell down in somebody's coal bin. I can't get out!"

Mario walked up the sidewalk and found the steps.

"Come give me a hand, but don't you fall in! It's nasty in here. I've got dust all over me."

Mario clicked his tongue. No sound bounced back. He wondered what happened to the house and why it was open to the cellar. He lay down on his stomach and felt for the edge.

"Here's my hand, Mario," said Arthur as he tapped his hand on some charred wood.

Mario reached down toward the sound and found Arthur's outstretched hand. "Give me your brooms first. Then I'll help you out."

With a mighty heave, Mario pulled Arthur from the dusty prison. "What happened, Arthur? How did you end up in that filthy old coal bin?"

"I don't know. I just walked up onto the porch and kept walking until I found the door. But there wasn't any door, and I just tumbled down. Ugh, my clothes feel dusty," he said while trying to brush off the coal dust.

Mario sniffed the air. "I think that the house must have burned down. I can still smell the stench of burned wood."

"You're probably right, Mario. Let's get out of here. Thanks for helping me."

The boys continued on their way. Arthur was more cautious than before when approaching houses, but the afternoon was still successful. They each earned $1.50 and sold all their brooms.

• ••
•

LIGHTING UP

SINCE GIRLS WERE not expected to make a living, they were not taught a trade. Girls were also not taught mobility; it was assumed that they would stay home. Only the boys learned how to walk with a cane and go out on their own.

Instead, the teenaged girls learned housekeeping skills, including rudimentary classes in cooking. At age sixteen, Jane was excited to finally get into the classroom kitchen. Her mother had always prohibited her from the family kitchen, afraid that she would hurt herself. But Jane was confident that she could learn to cook. She had to learn if she ever wanted to be independent. She knew that she didn't want to spend the rest of her life sitting at home on the farm. Jane was determined to live her own life and had begun to dream of a life with Mario. How exciting it would be for her to cook dinners for him every night!

Cooking class began with learning to use a gas stove. Divided into groups of three, the girls gathered at a stove in the home economics laboratory. They were allowed to touch every part of the stove; the girls learned where the knobs were located, reached inside the oven to feel how big it was, and examined the four burners. The teacher demonstrated how to light a burner: turn a knob, listen for the whoosh of the gas, light a match, and finally touch it to the gas. The girls with some vision tried first with varying success.

Jane was not anxious to try her luck lighting the stove. Fire scared her, and with no vision, she was afraid of burning herself. Just lighting the match was frightening, but after three attempts, she managed to produce a flame. Her hand trembling, she hesitantly moved the match toward the burner. The whooshing sound of gas changed as it exploded into fire, startling Jane. She jerked her hand, dropping the match into the flames and jumping back from the stove.

"Jane, you did it on the first try!" said the teacher. "That's very good."

"Thank you, but it's still scary," Jane said as she tried to stop shaking. "I wish that we had an electric stove. I read about them in *Good Housekeeping* magazine. They sound so much better than gas."

"Yes, electric stoves will be good for you girls. You won't have to worry about open flames and lighting matches. Most people still have gas stoves, especially in the country. Many of those houses are just now getting electricity, so it will be a few years before you'll find an electric stove out on the farms. You'd better get used to cooking with gas if you want to cook."

Jane wasn't comforted by the teacher's words. She knew that even though her parents' house would soon have electricity, her Pop wouldn't spend the money to buy a new electric stove. Even if he did buy one, Mother wouldn't allow her to use it. *Someday, when I'm married,* she thought, *I'll have my own electric stove and cook whenever I want.*

Jane learned how to read and follow recipes from Braille cookbooks. She memorized the graduated sizes of measuring cups and spoons; soon, she was able to quickly identify each size by touch. The teacher showed Jane how to hold a knife to chop vegetables, but Jane worried about slicing her fingers instead of carrots. She decided that once she had her own kitchen, she would not use knives. She would buy already chopped canned or frozen vegetables and fruit; she'd use kitchen scissors to cut up meat. She felt much more confident with the scissors and wouldn't have to worry about cutting herself.

Girls also learned to sew. Some wanted to make their own clothes, but Jane wasn't interested in such a difficult project. She learned to sew on buttons and mend rips, which were skills she would use for the rest of her life. She used a metal threader to thread the needle, but that was the easy part. The hard part was finding someone to help her to match the color of the thread to the clothing that needed mending. If nobody was around, she used white thread or waited until she could ask a sighted person for the right color. It was a constant reminder and frustration that she had to depend upon others to do things that sighted people took for granted.

After she mastered simple sewing repairs, Jane learned how to crochet. She quickly mastered the hook and enjoyed making a scarf. As an adult, Jane made many Afghans, dish rags, pillow covers, and baby blankets for her children and grandchildren. She knew what colors she wanted to use in each project, but of course couldn't shop alone for yarn.

* * *

Music stirred Mario's soul. At home, he listened to classical music on the radio, spending hours listening to Bach and Beethoven. Teachers at school played records to teach music appreciation; Mario looked forward to those classes with great anticipation.

Along with learning to play the piano and violin, Mario was required to master reading Braille music. After understanding the notes and the meaning of musical notation such as a whole note, half note, sharps, and flats, he needed to memorize each measure. He studied a measure, then played it. He repeated the process for each measure. It was hard work for him, and Mario wished that he could learn as quickly as some of his more musically inclined classmates.

Although he never felt very confident playing the violin, Mario joined the orchestra and was assigned the first violin position. He was also asked to join a piano quartet with three other boys, making for eight hands and two pianos; they memorized *Marches militaire* by Schubert, which they played at a school recital. The following year they played an adaptation of Tchaikovsky's *1812 Overture* at a school recital. Mario was saddened that his parents were unable to attend his recitals. Antonio worked twelve-hour days at the shop and Eletta was uncomfortable traveling alone on the interurban from Muncie.

While playing with friends was fun, performing a solo was another matter. Mario was terrified of playing alone before an audience. What if he made a mistake? Forgot the music? If others were playing with him, he felt less pressure and sometimes mistakes could be covered.

Mario vowed that when he graduated, he would never play a solo again. He was a perfectionist, never playing well enough to be satisfied, yet unwilling to make the extra effort to get better. It wasn't his passion. He knew that he couldn't make a living playing music. Some blind pianists played in bars, but the thought of trying to entertain rowdy drinkers caused him to shudder. His brother, Charlie, was already in college and talking about studying law at Notre Dame. Mario decided that he would also study law; he knew that practicing law was his only chance to earn enough money to someday marry Jane.

• ••
••

BALL STATE TEACHERS COLLEGE

WHEN MARIO WAS a senior in high school, he was already twenty years old and had been thinking for a long time about how he would earn a living. Staying at home with his parents for the rest of his life was not an option. He was in love with Jane, and he had to find a way to support her. He wanted to get married and have a family and a career. He wanted to be like everyone else in pursuit of the American Dream.

The school provided opportunities to learn a craft, such as caning chairs and making brooms, but the administration followed society's expectations that blind people generally could not make a living on their own.

Although Mario's brother was no longer living at home, the brothers remained extraordinarily close. Charles had attended Ball State Teachers College (now Ball State University) in Muncie for three years. Since a college degree wasn't required then for admission, he enrolled at Notre Dame Law School in the fall of 1933. Mario had idolized Charles since early childhood and decided to follow in his footsteps. He, too, would go to Ball State and then on to Notre Dame. He dreamed of practicing law with Charles in Muncie, earning enough money to get married.

On a Sunday morning in early October 1933, Mario sat with his parents at their kitchen table. They had attended the 8:00 a.m. Mass and were enjoying a hearty breakfast of Italian sausage and eggs. Mario would be leaving later that morning for Indianapolis, but first he had something to tell them.

"Dad? Mom? I need to talk to you about my future," he said solemnly. "I want to go to Ball State next year. You know how important my education is to me and how much I love to learn."

"Yes, son, we know," answered Antonio. "We've thought about your future a lot."

"But I don't have any money, and I'd need help paying for school. And I'd have to live with you."

"You can live with us," Eletta said. "I'd love to have you home again." She thought of how happy she'd be to cook Mario's favorite foods.

"We knew that the time would come when you'd want to go to college. We've been putting money aside, and there's enough to pay your tuition," added Antonio.

Mario brightened, smiling broadly. He was happy and relieved to have both financial and emotional support from his parents. Attending college would be challenging enough without adding money pressures. "Thank you, Dad. And Mom, I can't wait to eat your wonderful cooking every day!"

"What about Jane? What will she do after high school?" asked Eletta.

"She wants to continue her education at Ball State, too. Virginia [Charles' girlfriend] has already said that Jane can live with her. You know that Virginia lives just down Madison Street. We can all take the bus from here out to the college."

"It sounds as though you've figured everything out already. College won't be easy for you, but I know that you can do it," said Antonio. "It's almost time to walk down to the interurban station. Would you like some company?"

* * *

Senior year passed quickly; with graduation approaching, Mario needed help buying a present for Jane. He had no idea what a suitable gift would be for his beloved. In 1934, only engaged couples exchanged personal items such as jewelry or clothing. He wanted something special for Jane, but females mystified him. He decided to ask Charles' girlfriend, Virginia Pike, for help and typed the following letter:

Indianapolis, Ind.

May 21, 1934.

Dear Virginia,

Surprised? Well, you've guessed it. Won't you please do me a great big favor? There should be a five dollar bill in here which I'd like to have you spend for me. I hardly know just what might be appropriet for the occasion, but that is what your brains are for. You see, Jane is graduating this year, and I want to get something for her. Get anything but jewelery and clothes because we can't be engaged yet.

I'll bet you Had a swell time over in the east; I wouldn't mind going into those parts myself. It was mighty thoughtful of you to send me that card, all except the "ham sandwich" part of it because I was really hungry at the time.

> Do you know when Charles' school is out. We sure wish both of you could get here for the commencement somehow. Jane and I are planning a big private party that night and we'd like to have you with us. Just the four of us you know, like old times. Remember, I have ten dollars, a gift of the state, to spend.
>
> Well, don't forget to invest that five dollars for me, and heaven bless you for it.   Solong,
>
> Mario

Mario mentioned including five dollars in the letter for Virginia to purchase something "suitable" for Jane. Five dollars in the middle of the Great Depression was a generous amount; $5 in 2022 would be worth about $106. Likewise, the state of Indiana's gift of ten dollars would be worth $211. Mario was extremely frugal, and it was highly unlikely that he would spend the entire ten dollars on a graduation party, although they no doubt had a special dinner out.

Before he could celebrate, though, he had a final obstacle to overcome at the School for the Blind. He was summoned to the superintendent's office in early May and was informed that he had been elected valedictorian of his class.

"Mario, congratulations. It's a big achievement, and we're proud of you. As you know, the honor involves preparing a speech on a topic of your choice for Commencement," said the superintendent. "It should be no more than ten minutes long, and it must be memorized. You may not use note cards."

"Yes, sir," he replied, his heart already racing at the thought of memorizing and giving a speech in front of so many people. While pleased to win the honor, he was terrified of public speaking. What subject should he choose? How would he ever memorize it? What if he forgot the words?

With only a few short weeks until graduation, Mario had little time to decide on a topic, then research and write the speech. He thought about his father's immigration as a boy of twelve, traveling across the ocean to a new country with a neighbor—not even his parents. His mother came years later as a new bride, and although that must have been difficult, at least she'd been an adult. Immigration had played a very important role in his extended family, with several uncles and cousins having arrived in the States. He decided to speak on the history of immigration and began researching his subject.

At Commencement, the packed auditorium resonated with the excited voices of the graduates and their proud families. It was a hot June afternoon in 1934. During the Great Depression, the future was uncertain for everyone, both students and their parents. The economy had collapsed, and there were few jobs for anyone, much less young blind students. But that didn't diminish the joy of accomplishment for the students.

As valedictorian, Mario sat on the stage waiting for his turn at the podium. He wished that he had his note cards with him, though he had already memorized his speech; he could be going over his speech while listening to his classmate perform *Clair de Lune* on the piano. He felt sweat dripping down his face and wiped it away with the back of his hand. The music stopped, and he heard the superintendent introduce him.

He stood at the podium, cleared his throat, and began speaking the words he'd worked so hard to memorize: "My parents are part of the history of immigration in the United States." Nine minutes later he finished with a sigh of relief. He heard the clapping swell as the crowd rose to its feet and allowed himself a smile, acknowledging the applause. The ovation gave him some confidence, but it wasn't until a speech class in college that he was able to overcome his fear of public speaking.

Jane and Mario were the only students from their 1934 class of twelve students who continued to college. The rest went back to their homes. If the students lived near a larger town with resources for the handicapped, they went to work in a sheltered workshop. Others in more rural areas were forced to live at home and were dependent upon family for their survival.

In the 1930s, most women were not in the paid workforce. They were expected to be homemakers and raise children. Jane knew that she'd never work outside of the home and didn't need a degree. But she wanted to continue her education. When Mario told her about his plans to attend Ball State Teachers College in his hometown of Muncie, she seriously considered attending classes with him. Virginia, Charles' steady girlfriend, was also a student at Ball State. When she invited Jane to room with her and her father, Jane jumped at the chance. Instead of sitting and doing nothing at home with her parents, she would be living on her own and seeing Mario daily.

Classes at Ball State began in September 1934. Every day, Jane and Virginia rode a city bus to Mario's stop, where Mario waited for them. He lived with his parents only about two miles away from Jane and Virginia. When the three arrived at the campus, Virginia bade farewell and went to her classes. Mario and Jane walked arm in arm to their first class. Jane did not use a cane, nor did she ever want to have one. She felt incapable of walking alone and much preferred a companion to guide her.

Since childhood, Mario was fearless and often walked alone. On campus, he held a cane, but only to identify him as blind to others. He didn't swing it back and forth. That was unnecessary. He knew every bump on the sidewalks and how to find each building on the campus.

To orient himself, he listened for echoes of buildings or trees. He didn't worry about crossing streets, as there was little traffic on campus. Automobiles were noisy and easy for him to hear as they approached. Mario became so acclimated to the campus that he developed a clear mental map that enabled him to go wherever he wanted. Yet he couldn't let his mind wander while walking. He needed his wits to concentrate on his route or risk getting lost.

Mario was glad to have Jane as a classmate. Even better, they were finally beyond the scrutiny of the School for the Blind governesses. They could talk whenever they wanted, and enjoyed long discussions about their studies while relaxing over coffee at a local café. What a delicious feeling to hold her hand freely without getting into trouble with a governess!

As the only blind students on campus, Mario and Jane found it hard to make friends at first. Mario couldn't catch someone's eye to make contact. Someone would have had to approach him, and it seemed that most people didn't know how to talk to a blind man. He was glad to have Jane's company but longed to have male friends to discuss other classes and sports. Charles was studying law at Notre Dame, and Mario had become a big fan of the Fighting Irish football team. Jane listened politely while Mario told her about team statistics and exalted in their wins, but he missed having an equally enthusiastic partner to discuss the intricacies of Notre Dame football.

Since Jane didn't want to earn a degree, she took classes that interested her or would be of practical value. Mario was in both of her classes the first quarter. They took Principles of Geography and Ancient World History. Mario loved Geography and got an A, while Jane was happy with a B. Subsequently, she enjoyed additional history and typing classes. She liked typing letters to her sisters and also typed all of her academic papers.

One of the hardest things about school was keeping up with the reading assignments. Virginia was paid by Ball State to read to Jane, but Virginia had her own reading to do, so Jane had to wait until Virginia had time. Reading aloud took longer than reading a book by sight; Jane would have preferred to do her own reading, but there were no Braille textbooks yet, and tape recordings were decades away.

Mario, not personally knowing a reader, searched for one at the college employment office. He qualified for ten hours a week of readers. There were some federal rehabilitation funds available, so he didn't have to personally pay for their services. Many students applied for the thirty-five cents an hour job; Mario was allowed to pick the person who suited him best.

Jane and Mario took class notes in Braille, although it was hard to keep up with the professor. They used a slate and stylus, with special heavy paper inserted into the slate. Each letter had to be punched at least once ("a" is one dot) and sometimes up to six punches per letter.

Mario was proficient at making notes in Braille, but he would still be punching dots while the professor moved on to the next topic.

On days when he had a test, Mario lugged his heavy print type-writer to class. In one of his classes, the professor noticed that as the quarter wore on, an unusual number of students were getting As.

Some of his classmates had figured out that by listening to the taps of his typewriter, they could determine which answers were true and which were false. They copied his answers and got an A!

Jane successfully finished two years at Ball State, but in 1937, Virginia married Charles and moved to South Bend. With no place to stay in Muncie, Jane went back home to the family farm. Meanwhile, Mario stayed at Ball State for three years, and because law schools did not require a college degree in 1937, Mario applied and was accepted at The University of Notre Dame Law School. He was the first blind student to be accepted at the prestigious school.

Charles had already graduated from Notre Dame in 1936 and opened a practice in South Bend, Indiana. Mario was ready to follow in his footsteps.

After relishing her freedom, adjusting to life at home was difficult for Jane. Her sisters no longer lived at home. Irma was married, teaching school, and living on a farm about twenty miles away, while Ruth attended beauty school in Fort Wayne, Indiana. Jane missed her sisters. It was lonely on the farm with just her parents and no one her age.

Although Jane had received cooking lessons at school and was now twenty-four years old, Bessie still banned her from the kitchen. Every time she asked to practice her skills, her mother said, "No, the kitchen is just too dangerous for you."

She was allowed to make her bed and tidy her room, but Bessie was fearful that she'd break something and told her not to dust or clean the rest of the house. Frustrated, Jane spent hours reading Braille books. She subscribed to several magazines such as *Good Housekeeping* and *Reader's Digest*. Jane especially enjoyed the short stories and articles about current events. She also had a new Talking Book record player, which played recordings of people reading popular books. Jane listened to many books that she didn't have time to read in high school, including classics by Charlotte Brontë and Jane Austen. Reading helped to pass the endless hours on the farm.

Irma and Ruth helped to break up the tedium with occasional weekend visits home. Jane relished escaping the solitude of the farm, especially when her sisters drove her into Wabash, where they enjoyed shopping and trying on the latest fashions. On Sundays, Irma and Ruth went to church with Jane and their parents, then they all enjoyed a full Sunday dinner. It was hard for Jane when they left to resume their lives. She missed their laughter and stories; the house felt too quiet and accented her loneliness.

While neighbors stopped by to chat about farm prices or to exchange local gossip, Jane had no friends of her own. She was isolated both by farm life and her disability. Her only consistent link with the outside world was her parents' new radio, which used the newly installed electricity in the house. Rural Indiana didn't have electricity until the late 1930s, and both electric lights and the radio were novel and exciting. Bessie no longer worried about Jane accidentally knocking over a burning kerosene lantern. Every evening, the family sat under the bright light of two electric lamps and listened to news, music, and comedy shows. The radio provided an important connection to the world, and although Jane was still lonely, she could at least hear about the outside world and enjoy the music.

Letters remained her only way to communicate with Mario during his last year at Ball State, as the family still did not have a telephone. She read each letter multiple times, memorizing his words and trying to visualize his experiences. She missed their daily conversations from their Ball State days and longed to hear his voice.

Although Mario was only about fifty miles away, it seemed like a thousand miles. If bus or train service had been available, Mario undoubtedly would have eagerly traveled alone to the farm. But he was forced to wait until it was convenient for Charles and Virginia to drive him to the farm for a Sunday afternoon visit twice each summer.

∴

HANGING ROCK

JUST BEFORE NOON on a hot, hazy July Sunday, Jane heard the familiar rumble of Charles' old jalopy as it swayed over the rough gravel road. She leapt from the porch rocking chair and walked to the driveway, smiling in anticipation of a loving hug from Mario.

The couples spent a few minutes visiting with Bessie and Charles before heading out for a picnic at their favorite place, Hanging Rock. Only a few miles from the farm, Hanging Rock towered almost seventy feet over the Wabash River, appearing to hang over the river. Formed when the river undercut the base, the limestone rock had been used as a lookout point for Native Americans.

"Mario, if you'll carry the picnic basket, I'll take the blanket," said Charles, handing the heavy wicker basket to his brother.

"Sure, I'll carry it. Virginia, are you walking with Jane?" Mario asked as he took Charles' elbow to begin the hike up the rock.

"Yes, we'll follow you up. It's harder for us ladies to climb in dresses. But you boys go ahead and get a good spot," answered Virginia.

There were no steps, just a steep dirt trail littered with rocks and tree roots that seemed to lie in wait for Jane and Virginia to trip over them. It was a warm day. Both couples were sweating and out of breath when they reached the top. By the time Jane and Virginia arrived, the brothers were sitting on the edge of the outcropping, dangling their feet against the side. Virginia got upset when she saw them sitting there, terrified that they would fall.

"Charles! Get off that edge! Mario! Come on. You're scaring me!" pleaded Virginia.

The brothers turned and grinned. "Oh, Virginia, we're okay. Remember, we used to climb up to the top of the YMCA when it was under construction. This is safer than those steel girders!" said Mario.

"I know that story. You've always been crazy. Charles, please spread out the blanket and let's get some lunch," Virginia retorted.

Jane and Virginia emptied the basket, setting out the plates and silverware. Jane's mother had packed a bountiful basket of freshly fried chicken, deviled eggs, and potato salad. Bessie was a good cook, but Jane wished that she could have helped in the kitchen. It was hard to ignore the constant reminders that she couldn't do things that sighted women could do, but she wasn't going to allow that thought to ruin her day with Mario.

"This chicken is delicious, Jane. Your mother has really outdone herself," commented Mario.

Virginia looked up at Jane, who grimaced and said, "She likes to make it special for company. She has her own recipe, but she'll never teach it to me. I might burn myself."

If Mario heard the sarcasm in her remark, he ignored it. "And those deviled eggs are super. My mom never makes them, so the only time I ever get a deviled egg is when I come to visit you."

"Would anyone like more lemonade?" Virginia asked quickly.

After stuffing themselves, Charles said, "Jane and Mario, we're going for a walk. Do you want to go sit down by the river for a while?"

"Oh sure," Mario replied. "It will be good to get into the shade, and maybe we'll even dip our toes into the water!"

Charles helped the younger couple spread their old wool picnic blanket at the base of the towering rock, then said, "We'll be back in a while."

"Ok, thanks, Charles. See you soon." Mario helped Jane get comfortably seated on the blanket and then sat down next to her. Drawing her closer to him, she rested her head on his shoulder and relaxed in the peaceful setting. Cicadas sang their loud mating calls from the trees, drowning out any birdsong. The couple sat quietly as they listened to the sounds around them.

"Isn't it wonderful here, Jane? I can hear the water gurgling as it hits those rocks over there. It's quiet for a Sunday. I think that we're the only ones here."

"It's nice of Charles and Virginia to give us some time to ourselves. I like being down closer to the river. The shade is nice. Oh, feel that breeze? It feels so good."

"I'll tell you what feels good. Holding your hand feels good." "I miss you a lot, Mario."

"And I miss you. It won't be long now until I go to Notre Dame."

"I know. But I don't know how I'll make it waiting three more years for you. That's a very long time."

"Indeed. But we just have to take it a day at a time. It will be over before you know it.

And then we can get married!"

"Don't forget, you still have to prove to me that you can earn a living. I know that you can go to school, but earning a living is a bigger test."

"Jane, I'll do my best. I want more than anything to marry you and have a family. And I think that with Charles' help, I'll be able to convince you. I don't want you to live the rest of your life on the farm, but you'll have to be patient. I know that we'll make it." Mario sounded more confident than he felt. Both of their futures depended upon his ability to study, pass the bar, and make a living. Failure was unthinkable.

• •
•

LAW SCHOOL TERRORS

MARIO CLIMBED INTO his narrow dorm room bed and laid down with a heavy sigh. His muscles were tired but relaxed after swimming laps in the new gymnasium at Notre Dame. Every day he used an immense amount of mental energy concentrating on complex legal terms, but swimming in the buoyant water rejuvenated him. He'd enjoyed feeling free in the water ever since his brother Charles had taught him to swim years before in the old gravel pit. Keeping physically fit was important to Mario. He was a firm believer in the power of exercise to balance the constant mental concentration that functioning as a blind person required.

His brain was full of law cases that he'd studied that evening, and although he couldn't process any more complex information, his brain would not shut down. He had been in law school for two weeks, just long enough to realize the enormity of the challenge ahead of him. He tried to get comfortable, knowing that he needed to get enough sleep for the stressful day ahead of learning and memorizing complicated laws.

He wondered if it was after midnight. There was no glass cover on his alarm clock, so he could feel the position of the hands and know the exact time, but he resisted reaching over. The 6:00 a.m.

alarm would ring soon enough. It wouldn't help him to know that he had exactly six more hours of tossing and turning before starting all over again.

The nightly torment began. Thoughts ran quickly through his head in the long, quiet hours. Mario could not afford to lose his concentration during the day, but the familiar spiral of worry consumed every moment while resting. *What if I'm not smart enough? How can I learn all that I need to know? What if I fail? What else can a blind man do for a living if this doesn't work out? I don't want to make brooms or work the newsstand at the courthouse. I know that some blind people do that, and I'm happy for them. But I can't make any money and support Jane doing that kind of work! And if I can't support her, she won't marry me. Then what will I do? I'll be a lonely blind man living with my parents.*

I don't know how I can keep up with the professors. They talk so fast, and writing Braille notes is slow and cumbersome. By the time I understand what they're saying and get it punched in my slate, even with the shorthand I've developed, they've moved on to the next concept. Law vocabulary is full of multi-syllabic words, and there's no way that I can listen to the professor, understand, and write it down without getting far behind in a few minutes. God! I wish that I could take notes with a pen, like everybody else.

Mario felt his pulse quicken and cold sweat began to seep from his pores. He turned over onto his left side, trying to relax his muscles and stop the perspiration. Changing his position did not stop the thoughts marching through his brain.

And the amount of reading outside of class that they expect me to do! There's just too much! My classmates complain about how much reading is assigned, but they can read it themselves. They don't have to wait for someone to come and read to them. They can study whenever they want.

I have to depend on the schedules of my three readers, and that frustrates the hell out of me. They are nice guys, and I couldn't go to school without them, but they must do their own studying first while I lose time waiting for them. And listening to someone reading aloud is always slow; sometimes I think that we'll never get through the chapter. But at least I can type my notes as they read and keep up. They do enunciate clearly and willingly repeat a section when I ask. Thank God that Notre Dame pays for their services. I'm very grateful for that since I don't have any money of my own.

My Dad works long, 12-hour days at the candy store in Muncie to pay for my tuition. Mom helps there, too. What if I fail? They would have wasted all that money! They'd be so disappointed in me, especially after all the sacrifices they've made. I can't let Mom and Dad down.

He tried to cheer himself up by thinking about Jane's letter that he'd received the day before. His heart had skipped a beat when he reached into his narrow mailbox and found a thick envelope. It had to be from Jane! As he read and re-read her letters, he could hear her voice saying the words. How he longed to talk over the telephone with her. It would be so comforting to hear her voice. But even if her family had a telephone, long distance was too expensive.

Maybe I should try to study. Lying here isn't doing me any good. Mario sat up, reached over to his nightstand, and found a thick folder. Opening it, he lay back, propped against his pillow, and began moving his fingers over the raised dots. Reading the intricacies of contract law failed to make him sleepy. He memorized each point and tried to guess what the professor might quiz the class on in a few hours.

Finally feeling drowsy, Mario put down the Braille papers and closed his eyes. *I've got to get some sleep,* he thought. He turned over onto his right side, breathed out a long sigh, and tried to relax.

But thoughts of contracts and possible failure continued to float through his mind.

The sound of his alarm clock ticking away the seconds did not reassure him. Time was his enemy, pressuring him to stuff as much knowledge as possible into his brain. There was never enough time to master his classwork. Everything in his life took longer than for a sighted person. Every activity, from the time he got up until the time he fell exhausted into bed at night, required immense concentration. Getting himself dressed, shaved, and ready for the day took extra time as he reached for his clothes and hoped that he had no spots on his pants. His clothes, Braille books, and personal items were organized so he could remember where each was kept. Wasting time searching for something was extremely annoying.

Sighted students could walk to class without paying attention. But if he didn't concentrate and listen carefully for echoes while walking, he could easily get lost on the Notre Dame campus. How humiliating that would be!

Mario flipped onto his back and began taking slow, deep breaths. Concentrating on his breathing helped him finally relax. He drifted into a sleep punctuated by nightmares of becoming disoriented on his way to an exam and failing because of his lapse.

* * *

A chilly October breeze fluttered the curtains in Mario's dorm room, the only noise in the otherwise silent dorm. Friday nights in football season were usually quiet. The big game was Saturday afternoon, and the guys from the dorm were out celebrating in advance. Mario sat at his desk listening to classical music on his radio, feeling alone and left out. He wished that he'd been invited out with his classmates, more for distraction than for the alcohol. He wasn't fond of weekends. They emphasized his loneliness and passed slowly, something that his sighted colleagues could never imagine.

The next morning, he'd walk to the stadium with his tickets to the game. Notre Dame football tickets were coveted, so selling them was easy. Scalpers gave him $10, and he was happy to have some pocket money. It was impossible for him to follow the action without someone with him to describe the game; listening to the play-by-play on the radio made it much easier to follow the action and enjoy the game.

Mario rose from his desk chair and walked four short steps to his bed. Lying down with his hands behind his head, he listened to Tchaikovsky's fourth movement of Symphony No. 6 as it played on his radio, the slow tempo and swelling strings deepening his melancholy. He thought of Jane and how she was probably sitting at that moment in her favorite chair and listening to a Talking Book recording. She was so patient to wait for him to finish law school. It seemed like they were always waiting. Waiting for visits, waiting for letters, waiting for their lives to really begin.

He wished that he could share with Jane how anxious and overwhelmed he felt, but he didn't want her to worry. *She'll think that I'm not able to make it through school. Then she'll fear that she will be stuck living forever with her parents on the farm and be a spinster with nothing much to do. She'd be doomed to sit in a chair, reading Braille magazines and listening to time pass as the grandfather clock ticked the seconds and chimed each quarter hour. She's so isolated on that farm with nobody but her parents to talk to—what a horrible life that would be! I can't ruin her life by failing.*

I miss Jane so much. I wish that I could see her every weekend. Just holding her hand would be wonderful. How I long to hear her voice!

Mario sat up on the thin mattress and swung his feet to the ground. He might as well write Jane a letter and stop feeling sorry for himself. Sitting back down at his desk, he put a piece of thick paper into his Braille typewriter and began typing.

Gradually becoming more confident as the semesters passed, Mario began to relax a little. He developed two close friends, which helped to ease his loneliness. He enjoyed going to football games with them and discussing class homework assignments. He also joined a law student organization and participated in their activities.

By his third year, Mario knew that he would complete his studies. His grades were excellent, and he looked forward to graduating. The next hurdle would be passing the Indiana Bar Exam that summer. If he failed, he could take it again the following year, but he was already twenty-six, and their marriage would be delayed indefinitely since he would be wasting a year studying and not earning a living. With all the time and effort that he'd expended over the years—especially now that he was so close to convincing Jane that he could make a living and support her—failing the bar was unthinkable.

And yet, even if he did finish and pass the bar, Mario worried about how his blindness would be perceived to potential clients. He wondered who would want to hire a blind lawyer. He also considered the even more frightening thought that maybe he wouldn't be good enough to make money practicing law. Charles, who had moved back to Muncie, had asked him to join his practice. Mario knew that his brother would help him get established, but Charles could only do so much. If he couldn't prove to Jane that he could earn a living, she would not marry him.

Mario graduated *cum laude* from Notre Dame in June 1940 and was scheduled to sit for the bar exam in July. In some ways, his persistent worry pushed him to beat the odds. But his constant anxiety never faded. He knew that he would always have to work twice as hard as a sighted person. He had no choice.

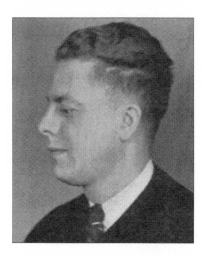

Notre Dame *Dome* yearbook photo, 1940.
He was the only student who appeared in profile,
thus hiding the empty socket of his right eye.

TAKING THE BAR

LAW SCHOOL HAD been predictable. Classes followed a comfortable routine, and Mario knew what to expect each day. He took his tests with a portable typewriter, as he had done at Ball State. However, he was the first blind person to take the Indiana State Bar Examination and assumed that one of the five board members would read him the questions at the beginning of the session. He'd transcribe the questions into Braille, then type the answers on his print typewriter.

The first session of the exam was held at 8:30 a.m. on a hot July morning in a hotel in downtown Indianapolis. Mario came prepared with his portable typewriter, a pad of Braille paper, and his stylus and slate. The examiners met him when he arrived at the testing room

"Mr. Pieroni, I am John Williams, one of your examiners. I see that you've brought a lot of equipment."

"Yes, sir. I have to be prepared."

"Well, Mr. Pieroni, you won't need all of that equipment. What we'll do is each board member will submit his set of questions to you and you can take the examination orally."

Mario was stunned. He was not prepared for an oral exam. His heart leapt, and he swallowed hard. It was one thing to demonstrate his ignorance privately on paper, but to face each examiner and have to come up with the answers while they were watching him made the task seem impossible. Yet there was no option but to go along with their plan.

"Oh, okay. Where shall I go?"

"We have a room just down the hall."

"May I take your elbow?" he asked, while shifting the heavy typewriter to his other hand. "Um, yes, sure," said the man. "How do you want to do this?"

"Just give me your left elbow. Then I can walk with you," Mario said while extending his right hand in search of the man's elbow. He hoped that the examiner wouldn't notice his shaking hand or hear his pounding heart.

Mario and the examiners settled into chairs facing each other. Although the tall hotel windows were open, it was stuffy in the small meeting room. The sound of passing traffic filtered in, and occasionally indistinct voices wafted in with the sultry breeze.

Mario felt as though he were at the Grand Inquisition; if he failed, his life would be over. He tried to get comfortable in the hard wood chair. He wished that he would have been treated like everyone else, but it was obvious that the examiners thought that they were doing him a big favor by allowing an oral exam. He took a deep breath in a vain attempt to slow his racing heart.

"Mr. Pieroni, as I mentioned before, my name is Mr. Williams. Are you ready?" He waited for Mario to nod his head, then said, "Here is your first question. Now take your time before you answer so that you're sure what you want to say."

Mario could feel Williams' eyes boring into him while he desperately tried to figure out the answer. He took another deep breath, hoping to calm his thoughts. *I know the answer. I can do this.* Finally, the words came to him. The questions continued all day, with a break for lunch. The same format occurred the next day, although each section had a different examiner.

Mario could not tell how he was doing. He couldn't see the examiners' facial expressions. He received no clues from their monotone voices. Each sat sphinxlike, uttering no sounds and giving no indication of a response to his answers.

At one point, Mario said, "So that is my answer, but I'm not confident about it."

"That's your answer, is it?" That was the first response from any of the examiners other than asking the questions.

"Yes, but I expect that it's wrong."

The examiner said nothing and went on to the next question. Mario was sure that he'd missed that one.

The ordeal ended late in the afternoon of the second day. Mario finished at about the same time as the others and stood in the hall, hoping to compare notes with his fellow examinees.

"Mr. Pieroni, we'd like to see you for a few minutes. Would you please join us?" asked Mr. Williams.

"Oh, sure!" replied Mario, not knowing why the examiners singled him out. Oh my God! Did I do so badly that they want to tell me right now to go home and give up law?" he worried.

He followed the examiner back into the same room and braced himself. He was surprised when he heard three different voices greeting him in a friendly tone. It was the first time that they had shown any interest at all in him.

"You know, Mr. Pieroni, that we of course cannot tell you whether or not you passed. You'll get a notice about that in about six weeks, but would you like to know some of the answers to some of the questions?"

"Oh yes! Thank you!"

As the examiners discussed a question from each section, Mario realized that the answers were the same as the ones he had given! His shoulder and neck muscles relaxed, and the overwhelming anxiety that had dogged him for years began to lift. Maybe he had passed after all.

After thanking the examiners, Mario left the room and made his way downstairs to the lobby bar, where he knew the other students would gather after the exam. He was surprised to be warmly greeted by many and realized that somehow the word had already spread that Pieroni knew the answers to the questions.

"Hey Mario! What was the answer to that question about the trustee distributing $10,000 cash?" asked one fellow, who pressed a drink into his hand.

Suddenly feeling very thirsty, Mario took a sip of a highball, cleared his throat, and began explaining his answer. While he was talking, he heard the shuffling of feet as others joined the crowd and felt the presence of others crowding around to hear him. One question led to another, and he dutifully repeated the answers he'd told the examiners.

Sometimes the group groaned and sometimes they clapped, depending on whether their answers were the same as his. Mario began to feel important and enjoyed "holding court" with his colleagues. His drink never went dry, and by the end of the party, things began to get hazy.

Later that evening, Mario went to a classmate's home to continue the celebration and enjoyed a "period of great exhilaration." The next morning, he woke feeling hungover, but the relief and joy he felt far outweighed the physical discomfort. He felt sure that he had passed, but still had to wait weeks for the confirmation letter.

Mario went back to Muncie for the summer to await the results and to prepare joining Charles in his law practice. The third week of August brought a letter from the State Board of Law Examiners of Indiana. He had passed the bar! Now Mario was ready to begin his career in the law firm of Pieroni and Pieroni.

Most of his mental demons had been put to rest by graduating and passing the bar. But he still needed to prove that he could earn a living and support a family before Jane would marry him. They did not want to be charity cases. Enough people had already told them that two blind people shouldn't marry, that they couldn't take care of themselves, or that he would be unable to provide for a family. The naysayers didn't dissuade him. Mario was determined to prove to Jane, their families, and the world that he could be a good provider. Jane was equally determined to prove that she could run her own household and raise their children.

With faith in his abilities and encouragement from Charles, he joined his brother and began the law firm of Pieroni and Pieroni on the top floor of the Johnson building in downtown Muncie. Shortly after he began practicing in September of 1940, a reporter from the *Muncie Morning Star* interviewed him. The article introduced the new lawyer and described him as having "a most pleasing voice, distinct diction, and a dignified bearing. The fair-haired, eager-faced young lawyer is well over six feet tall. He speaks of his blindness with utter lack of false constraint, putting himself and others at ease." The complimentary article provided a big boost to his business, as the phone started ringing with new clients.

That article would be the first of many photos and clippings that his secretary kept in scrapbooks. Mario, the blind attorney, was a novelty in Muncie, and the press followed him closely. As a result, he felt great pressure to be well-groomed and always alert. He never knew when someone would be watching him. That person could be a reporter, or simply a person on the street who would tell someone else a story about him.

When Mario bought his first Dictaphone, the company marketing department thought that he would make a great story to advertise their product. A company representative interviewed him and took a picture of him using the bulky machine. He could dictate letters and notes whenever he wanted, even when his secretary was busy. The Dictaphone and his Braille typewriter became indispensable tools. His secretary was available to read to him at almost any time, which was invaluable; the frustrating days of waiting for a paid student reader were over.

LEADING THE WAY

AS A YOUNG man beginning his law practice, Mario didn't want a guide dog. He used a white cane mostly to warn others that he was blind; he was able to get wherever he needed to go in Muncie without fear of tripping or getting lost. Mario concentrated on where he was at every moment, listening to the street sounds, and stopping at street corners. He did not walk with his arms outstretched. He was proud of his ability to navigate; but on rare occasions that he stumbled or tripped, he was embarrassed and angry at himself for his lapse of concentration.

Soon after Mario joined his brother in the office, Charles began encouraging him to get a guide dog. Charles thought that Mario's independence would increase with a dog, enabling him to navigate around town and travel on business trips more easily. After a few months of not-so-gentle nudging, Mario applied for a dog at The Seeing Eye, the first guide dog school in the country.

Jane never felt the need for her own guide dog but supported Mario's decision to get one. She was not trained to walk independently at the School for the Blind. Females, who were not expected to work or leave home, would always need an escort; independence training was only offered to the boys. If Jane wanted to leave the house, she depended upon walking with a sighted person. Being dependent upon someone else didn't bother her. She usually found a family member to accompany her on errands or shopping.

Mario took the train alone to Morristown, New Jersey, in early June 1941. Before the school would allow him to meet his dog, the trainers observed him for a couple of days. He had to prove that he was well-oriented and that he could walk around without assistance. Mario passed with flying colors.

Mario never forgot the day that he met Carla, a two-year-old German shepherd. She was a bright, spirited dog, and Mario took an instant liking to her. They were observed to ensure that the dog's personality matched his, along with her size and stride. When the trainers were satisfied that Carla and Mario were a good match, they began training with simple tasks. Mario learned to harness and leash Carla and how to feel her movement through the harness.

Mario trained with Carla for four weeks, learning how to work with and trust her. The instructors took them through any situation that he might encounter at home, such as low- hanging branches on a sidewalk, crossing busy intersections, and uneven sidewalks.

The trainers emphasized that it was a cooperative partnership between man and dog, stressing the importance of consistent discipline. He learned to reward Carla with lavish praise and affection every time she did what she was supposed to do. He'd pat her on the head and say, "Good dog!" He could feel her head looking up at him, and if they were stopped, she often licked his hand.

When Mario gave her the command, "Forward!" she took off at a swift pace. At first it was a bit intimidating to walk so fast with her, but soon he relaxed as he became more trusting of his guide. Mario, who was about six feet tall, had a naturally long stride, and the two walked well together.

It was important for Mario to concentrate while training. If his attention lapsed, he might not notice that he was at an intersection, or would forget to praise Carla when she did something right.

While out on the streets of Morristown, the trainer stayed with them and directed Mario which way to walk and which streets to cross. The trainer watched carefully for any potential problems or to correct his technique. Contrary to a popular myth, dogs can't see colors and don't watch the stoplight. The master is responsible for listening for the direction that the cars are going and to determine if they have stopped. The dogs are trained not to step off the curb unless it is safe.

Near the end of their training, Mario and Carla took the train into New York City for their ultimate test of managing in a large city. Blaring car horns and sirens echoed off the tall buildings, making it difficult to know if a car was honking at him or another car. Mario worked very hard to maintain his concentration as they threaded their way past sidewalks crowded with people, pushcarts selling hotdogs, and mothers pushing baby carriages.

Carla and Mario passed the test; he was so proud of her. He knew that if she could guide him through Manhattan, she'd be perfect to help him get around Muncie or wherever he'd want to go.

The new duo took the train back to Muncie, where Mario was expecting his parents to meet him at the station. He was flabbergasted to find not only his parents, but also a newspaper reporter. Carla was the first Seeing Eye dog in Muncie, and she was big news. The first of many stories about Mario and Carla was published in the local paper. Shortly after the article appeared, the Pieroni and Pieroni law firm telephone began ringing. Mario was pleasantly surprised to have several new clients in response to the publicity.

Immediately, he became even more recognizable around town. Mario was known as "the man with the dog," and people were eager to hear how a dog could lead a blind man to wherever he wanted to go. Over the years, he spoke to countless church groups, Boy Scouts, Kiwanis and Rotary Clubs, and students in high school and at Ball State Teachers College (now Ball State University). He talked frankly about his blindness, how the dogs were trained at The Seeing Eye, and how they helped a blind person.

Despite the number of talks and interviews Mario gave about his guide dogs, many people still believed that the dog knew where his master wanted to go and would take him there, stopping for red lights along the way. While it appeared to passersby that the dog was in charge, Mario was the master, telling the dog which way to turn. The dog only takes the master around obstacles and stops at curbs. Mario used his excellent sense of direction and concentrated while walking; if he didn't focus, or carelessly began to daydream, he could end up lost, the thought of which terrified him. It would be humiliating to be forced to ask for help.

On the street and in stores or offices, adults and children wanted to pet Carla. Mario had many opportunities to teach them not to pet or talk to her. He explained that Carla was a working dog, not a pet, and shouldn't be distracted. Gradually, though, it became easier, and people who saw Mario regularly learned how to behave around the dog.

The two quickly settled into a daily routine. Each morning, he put the leather harness over her head and belted it securely under her belly. The harness was critical, as it allowed him to feel every movement she made. That movement would direct him around people, sidewalk obstacles, and guide him to entry doors of buildings.

Double-checking that the harness was secure, Mario then attached her leash to the metal chain around her neck. With both in place, they were ready to head to the office.

Once Mario was seated at his desk, Carla curled up at his feet and waited for the next command. This was her time off, though Carla remained alert. If Mario needed to leave his desk, he simply attached her leash to the chair and said, "Stay!" The dog laid on the floor, patiently waiting for him to return. She was not allowed to roam loose around the office.

A few months later, Mario realized with surprise at how dependent he'd become upon Carla. She had increased his already strong confidence; now he could go anywhere and not worry about stepping into puddles or bumping into other pedestrians. An acquaintance told him that he made it look easy. He smiled and thanked the man but gave credit to Carla for being a dependable guide.

In 1946, *The Muncie Evening Press* ran a two-paragraph story headlined "Blind Attorney, Dog in Flight to West Coast." The article said, "Today he and his seeing-eye dog took off on their longest aerial jaunt to date—a trip to Portland, Ore., where the Muncie attorney is to appear in a legal action. Pieroni...left at daybreak for South Bend, where he was to catch a west-bound airliner at 10 o'clock." Traveling by plane in 1946 was becoming more common, but a blind man and his dog taking a trip by plane warranted noting in the local paper.

When traveling in unfamiliar cities, Mario often asked for directions, either from the hotel desk clerk or someone on the street and increased his already intense focus. Despite the challenges of walking with a guide dog, Mario and his subsequent seven loyal Seeing Eye dogs always found their way to his destination.

: :

GOOD ENOUGH

WHILE JANE WAITED seven long years for Mario to finish law school and establish his law practice, she had plenty of time to hear her folks' doubts about how they would manage as a married couple. Living with them on the farm provided her with opportunities to overhear conversations between her parents and other relatives. At that time, blind people were viewed as helpless, asexual beings who could not function independently. The very idea of two blind people marrying was unthinkable to most people. How could he earn a living? How could she cook and clean? There was no way for them to manage by themselves, much less care for and raise children. No doubt Mario's parents had the same concerns.

In addition to the skeptics, Jane and Mario had a more personal and formidable problem to overcome. Jane had been brought up in the Church of the United Brethren, a small conservative church in the village of Lincolnville. There were few Roman Catholics in her rural area; Mario was one of the first she'd ever met. He was the son of devout Italian immigrants who went to daily Mass and strictly adhered to church teachings. Catholics were only to marry other Catholics; both sets of parents worried about their child marrying outside of their faith.

Mario was also very strong in his faith and asked Jane if she would be willing to convert to Catholicism before their marriage. She agreed, although her parents made it clear that they disapproved of her decision. Her conversion was one more worry that Charles and Bessie had about the upcoming marriage. They were skeptical that the couple could be self-sufficient and didn't hesitate to relay their fears to Jane.

Yet Jane and Mario were determined to establish the life they'd dreamed of for so long. Mario worked hard to build his law practice and finally convinced Jane that he could support her. At age twenty-eight, Jane could plan her wedding and look forward to living an independent life with Mario.

Sixteen years after first hearing Jane's voice recite a poem in fourth grade, Mario and Jane were married on October 21, 1941. After the 8:00 a.m. wedding Mass held at Mario's parish church, St. Lawrence Catholic Church, the happy couple celebrated with a breakfast reception at a downtown Muncie hotel.

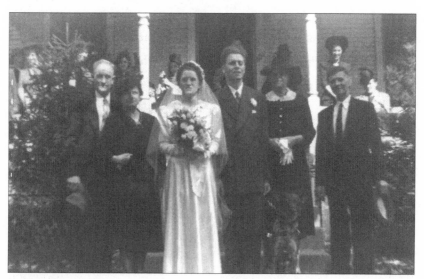

From left: Charles and Bessie Small, Jane and Mario, Carla, Eletta and Antonio

Jane's parents, sisters, and other relatives drove down that morning from their farms to Muncie for the ceremony. She'd been worried that Charles and Bessie might say something critical of her conversion and marriage in the Catholic church but was relieved that they were respectful and didn't complain that day.

Later that afternoon, Jane, Mario, and Carla boarded a train for Chicago, where they spent four days visiting friends and attending concerts. They stayed in the luxurious Stevens Hotel in downtown, which was quite the treat for Jane, as she had rarely traveled.

They had no difficulty getting around. Mario had been to Chicago on business several times and was familiar with the streets. One evening, they walked a few blocks to Orchestra Hall for a concert. If Mario wasn't familiar with how to get somewhere, they took a taxicab. When he needed directions, he asked the hotel's desk clerk. And if along the way Mario still needed help getting some place, he'd simply ask a passer-by.

Carla was an excellent leader for the couple. Before their wedding, Mario had taught her to walk with both Jane and him. Carla needed to learn how to leave enough clearance so that Jane, who walked on his right, would not bump into anything. Mario responded to signals from Carla, while Jane got her nonverbal cues from Mario by simply holding his elbow and following Mario's body up or down at curbs or starting and stopping.

Jane remembered many years later, "After a too-short honeymoon in Chicago, we took the train back to Muncie. That was the end; that was the beginning. It was the end of the romance and the beginning of our married life."

Married life was not as rosy as Jane had pictured it. Although Mario was busy practicing law, he didn't have enough money to rent an apartment. Eletta and Antonio offered them a room in their small, three-bedroom home on Charles Street, which Mario gratefully accepted. Jane wasn't happy about being dependent upon her new in-laws and hoped this would be a temporary solution. She longed for their own apartment, where she could cook and clean without Eletta watching her every move.

While adjusting to married life in her in-laws' home, tensions mounted in the United States as World War II raged in Europe. The U.S. had hoped to avoid being drawn into the War, but when the Japanese suddenly attacked Pearl Harbor only six weeks after Mario and Jane's wedding, the United States was thrust into the conflict. As the U.S. geared up for war, many resources were directed toward the military, which created shortages for the public. People became fearful that foods such as meat, sugar, and cheese would become scarce and began hoarding supplies. Food ration books were issued with complicated point systems. With Jane giving their allotments to Antonio and Eletta, there was usually enough food for the four of them, although careful planning was necessary. Having a sugar coupon didn't guarantee that sugar would be on the store shelves.

Eletta and Jane shopped often in the hope of finding meats or other staples. Jane enjoyed shopping with her mother-in-law. She got out of the house, and it helped to pass the time.

Although she used her daughter-in-law's coupons to help purchase the food, Eletta wouldn't allow Jane to help prepare it.

"I've always done the cooking, and I don't want anyone else in the kitchen. I know how to cook what Mario likes," she said with authority.

Eletta had no intention of allowing her to touch a pot or skillet. The rejection brought memories of how her own mother banished her from the kitchen. She was deeply frustrated that she still couldn't practice the cooking skills learned at school. Instead of feeling like a competent wife, Jane spent the late afternoons sitting in a living room chair, listening to Eletta clanking pans and smelling the aromas of dinner cooking.

Mario enjoyed sitting down in the living room with his parents after their evening meal, chatting about the day's events. Jane could either join them or retire to her bedroom. There was no other place for her to go in the house, except in good weather, when she could sit out on the front porch swing. If she wanted a private conversation with her husband, she had to wait until bedtime when they were in their room.

"Mario," Jane whispered. "Your mother won't let me cook, and today she told me that she will do our laundry. I can do the wash! She won't let me do anything around here."

"Well, that's Mom. It's her house, and she has her own ways," replied Mario softly.

"I'd do it her way. She fawns over you and ignores me. We're husband and wife! And I can't be a wife in her house."

Mario sighed. "It's only for a few months until I can save enough money for our own apartment. I thought that Mom would keep you company while I'm at work."

"I don't know if I can last that long. She's not much company. I hear her working all day while I'm doing nothing. It makes me feel bad that I'm not contributing. And today, she and your dad were talking in Italian so I wouldn't know what they were saying. I don't know if they're talking about me or about going to the store."

"I'm sure that they weren't talking badly about you."

"How do you know? You weren't there. Your mom doesn't like me. I'm so tired of being alone every day."

"Maybe you can visit with Virginia."

"She's busy with her children. I can't go to see her alone, and it's hard for her to talk on the phone with the little ones. I don't know anyone else. I can't get out unless Eletta takes me. I'm just stuck."

Mario sat on the bed, pulling on his pajama bottoms and yawning. "Well, I don't have an answer. Mom and Dad have done so much for me, I can't really say anything to them."

"Can't you at least tell them to speak English when I'm around?" asked Jane. Mario sighed. "I don't want to upset them."

"Well then, can we at least have more time in the evenings by ourselves? Your parents are always around, listening in, or you're talking to them. I miss talking just with you."

"Jane, my parents have sacrificed so much for me. All my life they've worked hard on their feet, making and selling ice cream and candy, just so they could take me to all those doctors to cure me. And when they realized that I'd always be blind, they saved for my education. They didn't take much for themselves. I owe them some time in the evenings."

Jane frowned and bit her lip. She wanted to say, "You owe me time in the evenings, too," but realized with a sinking heart that she'd never win that battle. His mother was always going to take precedence in their relationship; her husband was emotionally unable to stand up to his mother. On some level, Mario felt guilty about causing his mother so much suffering about his blindness. Even as a young child, he knew that her efforts to find a cure were all in vain, yet he had to obey her and submit to many examinations and treatments. Eletta was a too-powerful figure in Mario's life, and this unfortunate pattern for the marriage was set.

Every day was frustrating and humiliating for Jane. She felt like a child again, although now it was her mother-in-law telling her what she couldn't do. Mario had imagined that Eletta and Jane would enjoy each other's company and didn't realize how much tension had flared up between them. Jane knew that Mario wouldn't confront his mother, so she didn't tell him how tired she was of watching Eletta fawn over him, treating him like a child, while being snubbed herself. He couldn't see her face as she pursed her lips while Eletta indirectly, or pointedly, remarked on Jane's ability to function on her own. He didn't know how useless his wife felt day after day, or how criticized.

The stress of living with her in-laws combined with worry about the War accelerating and involving the United States left Jane feeling helpless and lonely. Mario worked hard all day, then came home and wanted to spend evenings visiting in the living with his parents. Jane was disappointed and frustrated that once again, her parents-in-law took precedence over her.

Mario was in demand as a speaker and was out several nights a week talking to church and civic groups. Mario enjoyed giving those speeches and rarely turned down an invitation to talk about his Seeing Eye dog or to advance the cause of blind people. But for Jane, each talk was yet another lonely evening spent listening to the radio.

His speeches were often covered in the local papers, including one talk in 1944 where Mario described what blind people were doing for the war effort. He emphasized that handicapped persons were making their own contributions and hoped that they wouldn't be displaced after the war with returning soldiers. It was a constant battle to educate the public and employers that blind people could work and be productive citizens, not just be dependent upon family or worse yet, beggars. There was no federal safety net in 1944 for the disabled. Some states paid a small monthly pension, but it wasn't enough for one to live independently.

One civic group that both Jane and Mario enjoyed was the Delaware County Workers for the Blind, an organization that provided assistance, social events, and help for over three hundred blind and visually handicapped people in the county. Mario served as president of the organization in 1941. While they enjoyed the monthly meetings, Jane needed more socializing and outside activities, yet with no telephone or transportation, she felt stuck.

Jane sorely missed her mother and sisters. Each day she eagerly awaited the mail, hoping for Braille letters from her mother and sister—their sole means of communication. His parents' telephone was used for local calls only; long distance was too expensive and reserved for emergencies or to relay bad news. Visiting in person was nearly impossible because gasoline was rationed. Jane's family drove sparingly and a trip to Muncie used too much gas. Antonio didn't drive or own a car, but even if he did, Jane wouldn't feel comfortable asking him to drive her to the farm.

She could only dream about the day that they would have their own home where she could cook and take care of the house without her mother-in-law's critical eye watching her every move.

FREE AT LAST

AFTER A YEAR of marriage, an apartment became available in a house that Antonio owned.

Mario and Jane moved in to the second floor of an old house that had been divided into two apartments. Jane was thrilled to have her own place. For the first time in her life, there was no one watching her, looking over her shoulder to make sure that she wouldn't hurt herself or that she was doing something the right way.

Jane read Braille cookbooks and taught herself how to cook. She'd learned the basics in high school, but that had been ten years earlier, and she hadn't been able to practice. Jane insisted on an electric stove. She'd never forgotten the frightening sound of gas and the prospect of having to light a match every time that she wanted to turn on a burner was too much. Jane also asked Antonio to make little notches in the dials so she could feel the nicks and know which corresponded to the low, medium, and high settings. She liked to use the oven, and with the temperature dial marked every twenty-five degrees, she learned quickly to make roasts and baked potatoes.

With Eletta's snarky comment, "You can't see, so how can you wash clothes and know that they're clean?" fresh in her memory, Jane set about learning to the do the laundry. That chore became a pleasure as she proved to herself and her skeptical mother-in-law that she could care for Mario.

Like most housewives in the 1940s, Jane used a wringer-style washer. It was in a small nook near the kitchen. She hooked up a hose to add hot water, added soap powder, and waited while the machine swished the clothes. The next step was running each piece of clothing through the wringer, putting it into the rollers while turning the handle to squeeze out the water. She was careful not to catch her fingers between the rollers, taking her time and concentrating on the task. Jane wanted spotless clothes; Eletta could be relied upon to point out any stains or dingy whites.

Jane took her heavy basket full of wet laundry out to the back yard, where she hung the clothes on a line strung between two trees. She didn't mind the clothesline in the summer, but putting on a coat and retrieving underwear and sheets frozen stiff as boards in the winter was unpleasant. On rainy days, Jane used a wooden rack set in the dining room to dry the laundry.

Jane taught herself how to iron using a modern electric iron. Mario's shirts needed to be perfectly pressed, or Eletta would be sure to notice. She smoothed out the wrinkles with her fingers, then ran the iron with her right hand while holding the fabric with her left. She could feel the heat from the iron before it got to her fingers; most of the time she maintained her concentration and avoided a burn.

Once they were settled in their new home, it didn't take long for the couple to think about starting a family. They'd always wanted children but were worried that they could be born with glaucoma. Visits to two doctors in Muncie convinced them that since there was no history of blindness on either side of the family, there was little likelihood that any children would be born blind. Both parents likely had recessive traits.

Jane was pregnant with their first child in November 1942 when she received a phone call with devastating news. Pop called to tell her that her mother, Bessie, had passed away. She had been ill but had been up and doing chores when she said that she was tired; she went to rest in her chair, but she never got up. Jane grieved that her baby would never know their grandmother. Indeed, Jane hadn't even told her mother of her pregnancy since she was waiting to finish her third month before announcing anything.

When their families heard of Jane's pregnancy, she could tell by their reaction that they wondered how in the world two blind people would be able to take care of a baby. Their doubt made her furious, and she wanted to shout, "I'm blind, not stupid!"

Jane also knew that the Muncie community would be watching. Mario was becoming well-known, and she felt that she'd have to be the perfect mother to prove herself. They were going to be held to higher standards than sighted couples. Jane knew that she couldn't see if the child's face was dirty, so she resolved to wipe her face after every meal. She bought extra baby clothes, enabling her to change the baby frequently and be confident that her outfits were clean. She didn't want people to say, "Oh, she can't see. She doesn't know that the baby is dirty. She's not a good mother."

Anne was born on June 8, 1943, a healthy baby with normal eyes. After a few days in the hospital, they came home to their little apartment and began life as parents. Like any new parent, they were attentive and quick to meet her needs. Jane hadn't been around many babies and certainly didn't have any experience changing diapers. She was terrified that she'd poke Anne; she would rather poke herself with the sharp pin. Jane used her left hand to hold the diaper away from the baby, and with her right hand guided the pin through the cloth to secure it. She pricked herself many times but never poked the baby.

Diaper changing didn't end with a clean diaper. Jane still had to pick up the wet, dirty cloth and put it in the diaper pail to be washed later. Disposable diapers were almost twenty years in the future, and she couldn't afford a diaper washing service. Jane cleaned them in the washer that required her to put each diaper through the wringer to squeeze out the water, then dried them on the clothesline outside in warm weather. In the winter, she let them dry on a wooden rack in the small dining room.

Mario wasn't much help with the baby; he couldn't change her diapers or give her a bath.

But he loved to hold her while Jane cooked dinner or did chores. Jane nursed for a couple of months and then switched to formula. In the 1940s it was considered more "modern" to use formula and bottle-feed your baby. While that opinion has changed in recent years, it was easier for Jane to have Mario feed Anne in the evening, which freed her to do something else. Mario enjoyed his time with Anne, cooing and making silly noises while she sucked at the bottle.

Late one afternoon after work, Mario climbed the steps up to the apartment. He stopped at the top to listen. He heard Jane in the kitchen. Anne was in her playpen, playing with a ball that rang a bell positioned inside. "Hello, Anne!" he said as he walked to the playpen. He picked up the ball, shook it and said, "Anne, come and get the toy!" She got up and toddled over. He could hear her footsteps on the pad, so he leaned over and reached out with his left hand and there she was! He went around to each corner of the playpen and repeated the game. Anne was laughing as she crossed on the diagonal, going from corner to corner. "Jane! Anne can walk!" he called out.

Jane stopped stirring the pot of peas and hurried into the living room. "But she's in her playpen. How do you know that she can walk?"

"Listen," Mario said as he shook the toy. "Anne, come and get the toy!" Laughing with glee, Anne obeyed.

"I heard her footsteps!" Jane reached into the playpen and pulled out her daughter.

Smiling, she said, "Well, now I'll really have to be careful. Pretty soon she'll be able to run away from me."

Aware that it was time to childproof the apartment, Jane put away anything breakable or poisonous and added a wooden baby gate to the top of the stairs. She was terrified that Anne would fall down the steep stairs.

Jane could hear her toddling around the apartment and know exactly where she was.

Occasionally, Anne got too quiet, and Jane would call her name. She'd laugh or make a noise, and Jane would go to her, reaching down to see what her hands were holding.

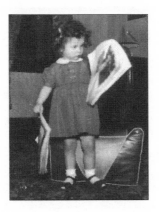

Anne at the Howard Street apartment

Two neighbor girls, who were about ten years old, came frequently to visit and play with Anne. They flattered Jane, saying that Anne looked like a movie star with her brown curly hair. One day, the girls asked if they could take Anne out to play in the backyard. They seemed responsible, so Jane agreed and allowed them to take her outside. Even so, she listened from the open window to make sure that she was okay.

The girls proved to be reliable, and Anne enjoyed playing with them outside. Once, on a cool, fall Saturday afternoon, the girls brought Anne home but forgot to close the gate at the top of the stairs. Soon after they left, Jane heard the most sickening sound imaginable. Anne was tumbling down the stairs, thumping against the wood in what seemed to be an endless fall. Mario and Jane were horrified. They ran down the stairs and found her crying but unhurt. Jane carefully checked her, feeling her head, arms, trunk, and legs. She couldn't find any sticky blood, and nothing seemed to be broken. Jane was too shaken to hold her, so Mario carried her back up the stairs. Moments later she stopped crying and began playing with her toys. She got over the fall a lot faster than her parents.

CONVENTION
ADVENTURES

FEELING MORE COMFORTABLE in his law practice, Mario developed an interest in local politics. When he began regularly attending Democratic Party meetings, one of the leaders noticed and decided that the bright young man could be an asset to the party. To encourage him, the mentor offered Mario a free one-day pass to the 1944 Democratic national convention in Chicago. The offer included a first-class train ticket, which sealed the deal for Mario. Fascinated with trains from his earliest blurry memories of steam engines belching smoke, he'd taken many train rides but had never been able to afford first-class fare.

On a humid July evening, Mario said goodbye to Jane and Anne, harnessed his dog Carla, and took a taxi to the Muncie train station. Passenger trains were common in the 1940s and were equipped with sleeper cars and elegant dining cars. The first-class section was at the rear of the train, lessening the likelihood that the engine's black smoke would enter the car through open windows.

He boarded the train to Indianapolis at 10:30 p.m. and made his way to the last car, hoping that it would be an observation car with an outdoor platform equipped with chairs and a place to stand.

Most travelers preferred to stay inside, but Mario wanted to experience train travel riding outside, feeling the motion of the train, and enjoying the sounds. He pushed on the last door, and to his delight, it opened. He found himself standing on the platform, the wind loudly rushing past his face. Too excited to sit down, he spent most of the hour and a half trip standing outside, leaning on the rail. He smiled as he listened to the turning of the wheels and the clanging of warning bells at the crossings.

Mario remembered his many previous train trips when he rode inside a regular coach. Although those seats were comfortable enough, he couldn't hear any outside sounds, only people's voices or the crying of babies. He'd been frustrated that he couldn't hear the clacking of the wheels or the powerful whistle. The air was typically stale, with cigarette smoke and cheap perfume assailing his keen sense of smell and sometimes giving him headaches.

The train slowed as they approached the train yards in Indianapolis. Gently rocking back and forth, the observation car bounced occasionally over switches that led to sidetracks, which were full of freight cars waiting to be coupled together to make a long train. Mario hung on to the railing, breathing deeply and even enjoying the sulfurous smell of coal burning. The brakes screeched as the train came to a stop. No passengers were moving to get off, so he knew that they weren't at the station yet.

A sudden loud whistle announced the imminent arrival of another train. He felt the vibrations on the platform and knew that it was going to be passing only feet away. When the engines roared past, Mario was thrilled to feel their immense power and size. The clanking, groaning, and squealing of the freight cars was thunderous. He was tempted to reach out and touch it but knew that was a bad idea.

Eventually, his train began to slowly move again. When they arrived at the station, a conductor directed Mario to the Chicago train waiting on a nearby platform. Now after midnight, he and Carla followed another conductor down the narrow aisle to his bunk. Berths were on both sides of the aisle, stacked two high. Mario was glad to have the bottom bunk, but it was barely wide enough for him to turn over and too short for his long legs. There was no room for Carla to sleep on the floor. He never allowed her to sleep with him but was forced to break the Seeing Eye's rules that night. Mario said, "Carla, jump up!" and she happily complied. He drew the thin curtain, which provided his only privacy, and tried to get comfortable sharing the small space with his seventy-pound companion. He smiled as the train's swaying motion train rocked him to sleep.

The next morning, the train was approaching Chicago, and Mario needed to get dressed. He found his clothes at the foot of the bed and, with some amount of effort, managed to put on his suit in the small space. He pulled open the curtain and stuck his feet out to get his shoes, which were under the bed. Carla got up and put her head on his shoulder.

A groggy male voice across the aisle said, "Oh my God, look at that elephant!"

Mario laughed and said, "No, it's just my Seeing Eye dog." He couldn't see the man's puzzled expression as he nonchalantly rose from his berth and walked with Carla to the dining car for breakfast.

When Mario arrived at the Democratic Convention in the Chicago Stadium, he felt his head almost explode with sensory overload. The auditorium was bigger than any Mario had ever been in, the noise reverberating in the cavernous space. A man shouted his speech into a microphone, which carried his voice, but from the babble of voices in the audience, Mario knew that few were listening to him. Delegates were talking and walking around, often bumping into him as he tried to listen to what the man was saying. Carla's head moved from side to side, but she remained calm as she worked to lead her master through the throngs of people.

That morning in the dining car, Mario had met a man from Richmond, Indiana, who was also going to the convention. Mario and his new friend spent the first two hours together as Mario got his bearings in the vast building. Navigating alone through the noise and crowds would have been very difficult, and he was grateful for a guide.

There was no doubt that Roosevelt would be re-nominated for his fourth term as president, so the delegates argued about the vice-presidential candidate. Roosevelt and his followers wanted Henry Wallace, who was Roosevelt's second vice president. But Wallace was much too liberal for many of the delegates. That's when Mario first heard about an opposing candidate from Missouri named Harry Truman.

Long debates dominated the day. When somebody opposed Wallace, the Wallace crowd booed and made ugly sounds, surprising Mario at how strongly people felt about their candidate. Experiencing the atmosphere in person was much different than following the proceedings at home on the radio. It became unpleasant for Mario to listen the rancor, and by the late afternoon, he'd heard enough. It was time to take Carla out for a walk and get some fresh air.

His return train didn't leave until after 10:00 p.m., so he decided to walk over to the convention's headquarters at the Stevens Hotel. He was familiar with the hotel because he and Jane had spent their honeymoon there three years prior. Mario and Carla wandered through the halls until he came to a ballroom with open doors. He stood and listened, hoping to hear the topic of discussion.

"Sir, would you like to join us?" asked a delegate. "We're the Texas Democratic delegation."

"Sure, I have a little time before my train leaves. May I take your arm?"

"You can sit next to me," the delegate said. "We're upset because we've been thrown out of the convention just because we're conservative. They say that something was wrong with our credentials, but that's not true. And we're mad. Real mad!"

Mario listened to the controversy and was appalled at the speaker's use of vitriolic language and anger. The man sitting next to him had seemed so pleasant, yet here he was yelling back at the speaker using even worse foul language. Feeling uncomfortable with the exchanges, Mario checked the time by pushing the small button on the side of his watch. When the lid flipped open, he fingered the watch hands and Braille numbers. Much to his relief, it was time for him to leave for the train station.

He enjoyed the cool night air and relative quiet after the raucous events of the day. He found the train station with no difficulty and boarded the train home. While a bit disappointed that the return ticket was only in coach, he was still able to take short naps sitting up. He arrived back in Muncie at 6:00 a.m., thoroughly exhausted, but with a new appreciation and appetite for politics.

CHANGES

ANTONIO HAD CLOSED the confectionery store in 1936, when Mario was finishing his pre-law studies at Ball State Teachers College. Tired of working long hours, he decided that he could make more money buying and renting out foreclosed homes in Muncie. As the Depression economy improved, he bought three lots in a newer neighborhood on West Jackson Street, only about three blocks from Charles' house. Antonio built two houses in the middle of the block, rented out the larger one, and moved into the smaller house next door. He moved one of his bungalow rental homes onto the third lot, which was on the corner of Jackson and Cole Streets.

Antonio offered to rent Mario and Jane that house. They jumped at the chance to have more space and their first house. Mario was thrilled to be closer to Charles, and Jane was happy for Anne to have cousins to play with. The house was small, but more importantly, it had a fenced backyard where Anne could play safely without Jane worrying about her running into the street.

In the spring of 1946, as Mario and Jane prepared to move to their new home, Jane learned that she was pregnant again. She was excited about the upcoming major life changes, but given her prior experience with Eletta, worried about living next door to her mother-in-law.

Being so close provided some benefits but also came with emotional strings attached. Eletta could watch from her windows or come over unexpectedly. Jane did not want to feel those critical eyes watching her every move.

Jane was frustrated that Mario had been unable to tell his mother not to interfere or criticize her. She blamed his lack of assertiveness on being "just too Italian," believing the Italian cultural stereotype where the mother is always right, and even grown men don't argue with their mothers. Further, she suspected that Mario relished being spoiled by his mother. Jane wasn't going to spoil him. She believed that he needed to do things for himself and spend time with her and the children.

Mario knew how much his mother worried about him and how many sacrifices she had made on his behalf. Eletta didn't have many outside interests; her life revolved around her family. Other than walking two blocks to St. Mary's Catholic Church for the daily 7:00 a.m. Mass, she rarely left the house. She spoke some English but wasn't comfortable in the language and didn't have many friends. Mario felt guilty if he didn't visit every evening with his mother, and while he knew Jane's preferences, he still chose to please his mother. His choice helped to solidify a lifelong smoldering conflict between the two women.

Moving into the new house took a lot of planning. Movers helped to pack everything, but they needed to be told where to put it once they arrived. Before the move, Jane and Mario went to the house and walked around, memorizing the layout. It was easy to decide where to place the furniture. The living room had a plain wall, with no windows or doors. The couch went on that wall, and the coffee table went in front of the couch. They always had to remember that it was there, since the table's sharp edges bruised their shins if they misjudged or forgot about its location.

Eletta helped Jane shop for new curtains. She described the colors and patterns of the fabric while Jane felt each fabric sample. Jane tried to visualize what the design looked like as Eletta took her hand and ran it over the pattern to show Jane how big it was. It must have been frustrating to rely on her mother-in-law's opinion, but Jane made the final decisions.

Having their home look as normal as possible was very important to the couple. They put pictures of Anne and some landscapes on the walls. They turned on the lights when it began to get dark, and Mario turned them off when it was time for bed. Although he had a very small amount of light perception, he also lightly touched the bulb to check for heat, which indicated that the bulb was on. He didn't want to turn on a bulb that should be off. Anne, of course, needed the lights at night. And they wanted people to know that they were home. If it were dark inside, friends might assume that nobody was there.

Although Jane did almost every chore in the home, she refused to feed coal to the basement furnace. Throwing coal into a hot fire was a dirty and dangerous task which Mario undertook with enthusiasm. He couldn't fix things around the house like many other husbands, but he could keep the home fires burning.

"Anne? Would you like to come down into the basement with me and watch me put coal into the furnace?" asked her father. "We need to add more coal now because if we don't, this house will get mighty cold!"

"Yes! I want to see the fire!" Four-year-old Anne was not allowed in the basement without an adult, and she was excited to have the opportunity to go down with her dad.

Anne and Mario felt the air become damp and cool as they descended the wooden steps. It was dark, with only a dim light bulb and a window at ground level to provide a sliver of light. The furnace seemed huge, with ducts that resembled octopus tentacles reaching up towards the ceiling.

Mario opened the furnace door. Heat rushed out, and Anne took a step back. "Oh! It's really hot."

She watched as her father slowly pulled on a pair of heavy gloves and picked up a handful of coal from the bin. The hot flames danced inside while he tentatively felt for the opening and threw in the coal.

"Dad, aren't you scared?"

"Well, I'm careful. I can feel how hot it is and the gloves keep my hands from getting burnt. I can hear the coal as it lands in the furnace, so I know that I threw it in the right place. I use gloves because I can't keep the coal from sliding off the shovel. It's easier for me to just pick it up. Here, I'll throw in some more coal. There! Can you hear it?"

Anne peered around her father and winced as the flames grew higher. "Yes, but it's scary

Can we go back upstairs now?"

"Sure. It's important that I don't let the fire go out. It would get awfully cold in the house, and I couldn't get it started back up again by myself. Your grandpa would have to come over, and it's a lot of work, so he wouldn't be happy. I'll be back tomorrow morning and put some more coal in."

Anne ran to the stairs, happy to leave the furnace monster behind. Several years later, when the nuns at St. Mary's talked about the fires of hell, she got the picture.

* * *

Anne was good at entertaining herself, but Jane felt that she needed more than what she could provide at home. When Emerson Country Day School offered Anne a scholarship, Jane and Mario immediately accepted. It was considered an excellent preschool, and although only three blocks from the house, they had no way to get her there. Mario worked in the opposite direction, and Jane never walked anywhere outside the home unescorted. Eletta did not volunteer to walk her granddaughter to school, so Jane and Mario decided that at age three, Anne could walk to school by herself. They taught her how to cross the quiet side streets, and when she arrived at busy Tillotson Street, the son of the school's owner met her and helped her to cross. In 1946, there was little traffic, and nobody worried about strangers kidnapping their children.

Anne enjoyed walking to school, feeling safe as she waved to neighbors protectively watching her from their porches. Jane stood at her front steps, listening for her cheerful, "Bye Mom! I'm across the street now!"

With a smile and a wave, Jane called after her, "Be careful crossing the next street. I'll see you at lunch time."

After walking past several houses, Anne came to the Cardinal Shop. She always paused to look at their windows full of toys, books, school supplies, and dolls on display. Next door was Ray Keesling's grocery store and restaurant. Ray knew the Pieroni family well and kept a running tab so when the children grew older, they could go and pick up grocery items for their mother.

Across the street from Keesling's was a wooded lot that Anne especially enjoyed passing. Violets covered the ground every spring, and Anne liked to bring home little bouquets for her mom. It didn't matter what the weather was like; even tromping in the snow was fun as she watched the tracks her boots made. Anne never complained about the walk. Nursery school was fun, and there was always something interesting to see on the way.

Jane delivered their second child, John Charles, on December 31, 1946. She found that caring for him was easier, since she knew more of what to expect, and was much more experienced with diapers and bottles. Anne was three and a half and excited to have a baby brother. As he grew older, she entertained him with toys and let Jane know if he was getting into something he shouldn't. Anne learned very quickly, though, to put away the toys and to never leave anything on the floor where her parents could trip over it. If Jane walked into the living room where she was playing on the floor, she warned her mother and Jane walked around her.

Mario and Jane relaxed by reading the Braille editions of *Reader's Digest* magazine. Jane also enjoyed *Ladies Home Journal* and *Good Housekeeping*. Mario read more scholarly journals, including *America,* which discussed events and controversies in the Roman Catholic Church. Although they couldn't read print books or magazines, it was important that they set a good example for their children.

Most of the time, Jane had no regrets about being a blind mother. But while tucking her children into bed at night, she always wished that she could cuddle next to them and read a story. Braille children's books didn't exist then, and even if they had, the experience would have been very different. Since there are no pictures in a Braille book, a sighted young child would be bored staring at Braille dots. Half the fun of reading a picture book is talking about the illustrations, something that is lost if the parent can only finger the words.

Between nursery school and Mario often asking her to spell the words on signs or on cereal boxes, Anne learned the alphabet and simple words. It wasn't surprising to Mario and Jane that Anne learned to read at a very early age. She brought home books from school and read the new children's magazine, *Highlights*, from cover to cover as soon as it arrived. Later, when Anne was in elementary school, they subscribed to the print editions of *Reader's Digest*, *Saturday Evening Post*, and *Life* magazines.

Mario often asked Anne to describe what she saw around her. He did it partly to orient himself, but mostly it was a way to increase her vocabulary. On evening walks with Anne, he'd ask her to read letters from signs and then tell her the word. She might tell him about the white house with the big tree in front, and if the tree were close to the sidewalk, they'd stop and put their arms around it to see how big it was.

"My! That's a big tree. It must be very old. I can't even reach all the way around it. Can you?" Mario reached down to feel Anne's arms as she stretched to hug the tree. "Oh! I see that the tree is too big for you, too. You'll have to grow very long arms to hold this tree!"

Anne laughed and stopped at many big trees on their walks.

One summer night, when Jane and Mario were sitting out on the front porch swing, Mario asked Anne, "What do you see in the sky tonight?"

"There is a moon," she answered. "How does it look?"

"Tonight," she said, "It is all put together."

⠒⠂

QUICK-WITTED

WHEN THEY WERE married, some people—including their relatives—didn't think that two blind people could manage. Who would take care of them? How could they raise any children by themselves? Jane was determined to keep both her house and children clean. What would people say if her children wore dirty clothes? That poor blind Mrs. Pieroni doesn't know that her children are dirty? She must not be fit to raise them. Jane feared that child welfare would decide that she was an unfit mother because of her blindness, so she made sure that her children always wore clean clothes and went out with washed faces. One spot on a blouse did matter.

As Anne grew older, Jane asked her to check everyone's clothes for spots. "Anne, do I have any spots on my dress? How about Johnny's pants?"

Jane bought play clothes for each child, along with school clothes and Sunday outfits. It was easier to keep the nicer clothes for dress occasions, and she worried less about spots on the play clothes. She knew that children need to play and would get dirty, but they must put on clean clothes the next day. Likewise, Jane had housedresses that she only wore around the house. She always wore an apron, which saved her dress from a lot of food spills. But whenever she went to the grocery or anywhere out in public, Jane changed into a good dress fresh from the laundry that she knew was spotless.

Despite the naysayers, Jane proved to be a competent mother. She did all the diapering, washing, cooking, feeding, cleaning, nursing, and shared disciplining with Mario. But there was one thing that Jane couldn't do for her children. She couldn't cut their fingernails.

When Anne was a very young baby, Jane tried to cut her nails with a small pair of scissors. She cut too deeply, making the finger bleed and Anne cry out in pain. Jane felt terrible and resolved to ask a sighted person for help. Her sister-in-law, Virginia, had four children; Jane reluctantly asked her. Virginia stopped by the house occasionally and trimmed them for her. Jane was grateful but wished that she could do it and not be forced to rely on someone else. When Anne was old enough to cut her own nails, it became her job to trim her younger siblings' nails. She didn't complain about the extra chore, although every time Anne got the scissors and sat down with John, Jane felt a stab of sadness that she couldn't perform such a simple task.

* * *

Jane trudged up the wooden basement steps, a heavy basket of wet sheets propped against her hip. Eighteen-month-old John followed closely behind, hanging onto the hem of her skirt. It was a warm spring day, perfect for drying the load of sheets. She didn't yet have a dryer, and used the clothesline strung across the back yard to dry their laundry.

"Johnny, I'm going to hang these sheets up. You come with me outside. Go find your truck!"

Jane heard his little shoes running on the sidewalk, then stop when he found the truck. She listened as he imitated truck sounds and rolled the red metal toy on the cement. Jane set about picking up the sheets and fastening them to the line with wooden clothespins. Minutes later, she realized that she didn't hear her son anymore. "Johnny? Where are you? What are you doing?"

When he didn't answer, Jane became alarmed. Trying not to panic, she called again, a note of fear in her voice. "Johnny! Answer me!"

Seconds later, Jane heard the toddler giggle. It sounded as though he was over by the Cole Street fence. Ducking under the clothesline, Jane walked toward the fence, hoping that he was still inside the yard.

"Johnny? Where are you?" Jane tried to keep her voice calm while hoping that his answer would guide her to him. She reached the fence and to her horror, found that the gate was open.

How would she find him now? He could be anywhere, or worst of all, in the street that was only feet away.

Jane's heart was pounding. She knew that if she tried to chase him, he'd just run into the street and away from her. Jane stood still for a few moments, then said, "Well Johnny, I have to go in. I'll leave the gate open. You can come in when you're ready." She turned around and walked back into the house. When he saw her go inside, he had no interest in staying out alone.

Much to her relief, Jane heard the tapping of his little feet as he ran on the cement sidewalk toward the back door.

"Mommy? Where are you?" called the toddler.

"I'm right here, Johnny," she said as she opened the screen door for him.

Deliberately going off and leaving a very young child by the street was the hardest thing that she'd had to do as a parent, but it was the only way she knew to get him back inside to safety.

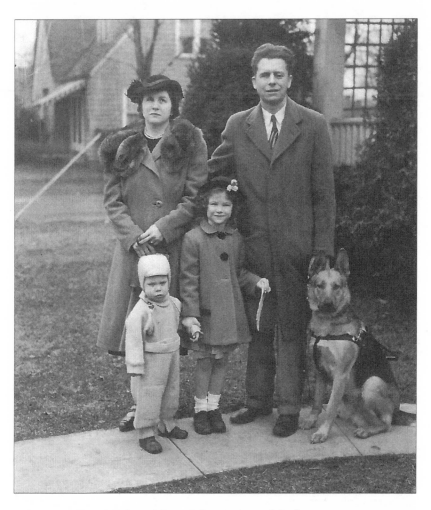

Jane, Mario, John, Anne, and Carla

∶ ∷

CAN'T WIN

ANNE AND JOHN were healthy, but like other children, they sometimes became ill with childhood sicknesses such as measles and chicken pox, which were not preventable by vaccine in the 1950s. Jane didn't need a thermometer. She could tell by touching the child's forehead and body if they had a fever. Unusually cranky behaviors were another clue that something was wrong. She gave extra fluids and rocked the sick one to sleep while waiting on their pediatrician, Dr. Young, to stop by the house after office hours. While there was little that he could do to cure an illness, it was comforting to hear his reassuring words.

When the children were very young, Eletta often accompanied them on the bus to Dr. Young's office for regular checkups. Jane never left the house alone and needed Eletta to help her navigate while managing two children. But when Anne turned five, Jane realized that she could walk with Anne and hold two-year-old John's hand. She didn't need her critical mother-in- law to go with her. Anne was a careful guide, and Jane felt safe with her.

Riding on the bus to Dr. Young's office for an appointment, Anne became aware of two women staring at them. She heard them talking about her mother.

"Well, at least the children can see. How does she manage?"

"I can't imagine. She must have a lot of help."

"There's no way she can do it alone. How can she change diapers? What if that cute little boy runs away from her? She'd never be able to catch him."

"And he could get hit by a car!"

"I know. They look pretty clean. How does she know if they're dirty?"

Anne looked at her mother's face. She could tell by the way that her lips were pressed together that her mother was angry to be talked about as if she were also deaf and stupid.

Minutes later, the bus came to their stop and with relief, the family got off. Anne was angry for her mother and never forgot the overheard conversation.

* * *

Although they lived next door to Mario's parents, Jane did not want to depend on them for babysitting or help with the children. She rarely took them for visits, although as they got older, they often went by themselves to Grandma's for Cokes or candy. Jane never bought soft drinks or kept much candy in the house, so the children considered it a great treat to run next door for the forbidden sweets.

The extra calories eventually became a problem when John was eleven and was gaining too much weight. Jane asked Eletta to stop giving him the treats, but she refused. Jane was furious. She complained to Mario, who explained that Italian mothers like to spoil their sons. Jane didn't buy that explanation but was powerless, knowing that he wouldn't confront his mother.

Eletta further offended Jane when she criticized Jane's new hairstyle. She was deeply hurt, yet when she told Mario, he replied, "That's the way she is. She doesn't ever go to the hair salon. I don't think that she's ever cut her hair." His explanation did not mollify Jane.

When men's wash-and-wear shirts became available, Jane was thrilled. She wouldn't have to spend so much time and energy ironing. Eletta did not approve of permanent-press clothing and implied that she was not being a good wife if she didn't iron Mario's shirts. Jane was not pleased with her implication but didn't argue. Her resentment toward her critical mother-in-law grew, and while Jane rarely argued with Eletta, she also never forgot the painful barbs.

Much as she disliked depending upon her mother-in-law, Jane still needed some help with the grocery shopping or buying clothes. One cold January day, Eletta and Jane took five-year-old Anne and two-year-old John out shopping. When they arrived home, John had a dirty diaper and Jane was in a hurry to get him changed. Anne took off her coat while Jane quickly pulled off John's little blue coat and handed it to Eletta.

Jane carried John into the bathroom, and Eletta hung the coat to dry on a wall sconce with a hot electric light bulb and went into the kitchen.

Minutes later, smoke began curling from under the coat. Jane dashed into the living room, frantically calling, "I smell smoke! What's burning?"

Anne looked up and saw a flame pop out from the coat. "Johnny's coat is on fire!" Astounded, Anne stood back as she watched Eletta grab the coat, throw it to the floor, and stomp out the fire.

Jane was angry and frightened. "How did it catch fire?" she demanded, frowning in Eletta's direction.

"I thought that it might dry faster on the light bulb. I didn't think that it would catch fire!" said Eletta.

"How could you do that? You're an adult! You should have known better than to hang that coat over a light bulb!" Jane said as she reached down to pick up the coat. The smell of burning wool still hung in the air. She fingered the material, finding a large hole. "It's ruined. I'll have to buy another one," she said with a disgusted tone. "You could have burnt the house down. You scared me to death when I smelled the smoke." Shaking her head and with her heart still pounding, Jane turned and said, "Anne, you play with John while I finish cleaning up the bathroom."

Later that night, Jane told Mario about the near disaster. "Now Jane, don't be so hard on her. Mom was just trying to help. She put out the fire. No harm done."

"Don't placate me! You weren't there. If the house had burned, they'd have said that the blind woman caught her house on fire and we're not fit to raise those kids. I have to worry about things like that. Your mother didn't. She could see, and nobody would have criticized her. And now I'll have to buy John another coat. I doubt that she'll pay for it, and she knows that money is tight for us. It just makes me so mad."

Mario heaved a loud sigh, and said, "I don't know what I can do. It doesn't seem like I can please either of you."

"I feel as though everything I do is graded, and nothing that I do measures up to her expectations. I can't relax around her, Mario. I always have my guard up. She watches everything that the kids or I do. She doesn't hesitate to let me know that I'm deficient in many ways. What can I say back to her? She's my mother-in-law, and I can't argue with her. I just bite my tongue and try not to spend any more time with her than I have to. I do appreciate that she helps me shop and will babysit if I absolutely need a sitter, but you know I don't like to ask her. I don't want to owe her any favors."

Eletta never offered to buy a new coat for John, and Mario didn't mention the incident to his mother. Tensions between the two women continued. Jane rarely invited Eletta and Antonio over for dinner, and the family went next door to celebrate Easter or other special occasions only when Charles and his family were there. Eletta did not stop by for informal visits or coffee, although Antonio occasionally went over to fix something at the house. Mario continued his nightly visits, irritating Jane, who would have appreciated help with baths and getting the children into bed.

Jane had no one nearby to provide emotional support, and few close friends. Her own mother had died just before Anne was born, and her sisters lived over an hour away. She couldn't telephone Ruth or Irma, as long distance was typically used only for emergencies or to spread big news, not to let off steam. She didn't feel comfortable writing about her problems in letters to her sisters. The letters weren't private, and by the time she had a chance to write, her anger had cooled off. Jane stuffed her feelings and continued to bite her tongue. But the suppressed anger and resulting stress would come at a price to her body, as later she developed chronic illnesses that caused unrelenting pain.

GLASS EYES

SHORTLY AFTER NOON, on a cool spring day in 1947, Jane heard small footsteps running up the front steps and the front door slam. She sighed with relief. Anne was safely home from preschool. Although Anne was now four and had been walking alone to and from the school for a year, Jane still wished that she could accompany her. It was yet another example of something she couldn't do for her child. But walking alone didn't seem to bother Anne. She cheerfully left the house every morning and happily returned in time for lunch.

"Hi, Anne, how was your day at school?" asked Jane as she helped remove Anne's red sweater

"It was okay," she replied. Anne looked up at her mother's face and studied her eyes as if for the first time. "Mom, why is your eye so big?"

"My eyes were sick when I was born. One eye just got a lot bigger. Why do you ask?"

"Nancy said that your big eye was ugly and scary. She wanted to know why it was so big. I told her to leave me alone."

"Oh dear! I'm sorry that happened. Don't pay any attention to her."

"Nancy is stupid. What's for lunch?"

While Anne didn't appear to be emotionally upset by the classmate's question, Jane was embarrassed and horrified that her daughter was already being teased. She didn't want Anne to suffer because of her blindness, or the appearance of her eyes.

Jane remembered looking into the bathroom mirror as a young child. With the limited vision that remained, she had stared at her bulging eyes, hating them. She ignored her fair skin, rounded chin, plump cheeks, and short brown hair, convincing herself that her swollen eyes made her ugly. She stared at her fuzzy reflection, angry that she could do nothing to change it. Her classmates teased her and told her that someday her eyes would pop out of her head.

Whenever she was out in public, even with faint vision, she could still see people staring at her. Jane felt ashamed of her eyes, and was embarrassed to be singled out.

As an adult, completely blind, she felt the stares and endured hearing whispers about her appearance. Jane wanted to look like a normal woman. She had tried to hide behind a pair of eyeglasses and even wore them for her high school graduation picture. Later, she admitted to herself that people could still see her misshapen eyes through the clear lenses. She stopped wearing the glasses; she was only fooling herself.

Ever since Jane had read that it was possible to remove her eyes and replace them with artificial glass eyes, she had longed for the day when they could afford the surgery. Mario, while supportive of her desire to get glass eyes, always worried about having enough money to pay for the operation. She vowed to wait no longer. Jane decided that afternoon to have the surgery. The first child at school had asked questions and there would be others. It was time to be rid of the offending eye. Perhaps she could save money by having only her largest eye removed—it would be better than nothing.

She found a doctor in Indianapolis who suggested that both eyes be removed. He told her about artificial glass eyes and how they would make her look normal. She could even choose the eye color! Jane was excited about the prospect and anxious to have the operation. She scheduled the surgery for the following month.

Jane was surprised when Eletta offered to take care of Anne while she was in the hospital and gratefully accepted. In the mid-1940s patients were routinely hospitalized for at least a week after surgery. Jane didn't mind being in the hospital for that long. She enjoyed the rest and not having to worry about cooking or doing the housework.

After she had recovered from the operation, Anne, Mario, and Jane took the train to Chicago for her appointment to be fitted for her first pair of artificial eyes. Anne was fascinated by the rows of glass eyes lined up neatly by color on trays. She stared at the unseeing eyes and felt a shiver, yet was fascinated by the many sizes and shades of brown, blue, and green looking up at her. She anxiously watched the man work to get the correct eye size for her mother. Jane's relaxed and calm demeanor comforted Anne. This was simply the next step to fulfilling her mother's dream, and no pain was involved.

The man asked Jane what color eyes she wanted. She paused while trying to visualize what she would look like with brown, hazel, or blue eyes. Sensing her hesitation, he suggested, "Why don't you get blue eyes to match your daughter's pretty eyes?" She accepted his advice, relieved to have made the decision. Anne felt special that her eyes would match her mother's.

Jane was thrilled to finally feel that her appearance was much more like a "normal person." She hoped that strangers would no longer ask her bluntly, "What happened to your eyes?" She was tired of telling them that she was born with glaucoma, while knowing that it was none of their business. People might watch her, knowing that she was blind, but now that her eyes looked normal, she shouldn't attract pitying looks or rude comments.

Happy with the outcome, Jane told Mario that he, too, should have the operation. She knew that his big left eye was ugly; surely people stared at it like they had at hers. But Mario said no, allowing no further discussion. He absolutely would not consider glass eyes. Jane was disappointed and brought up the idea many times over the years, but he refused to change his mind. She never understood why he wanted to keep his eye, maintaining that he could have greatly improved his appearance.

Perhaps if Mario had been more forthcoming with his memories of his traumatic childhood surgery, Jane could have been more sympathetic. For Mario, the unusual appearance of his eyes was a small price to pay for sensing even a bit of light. During his lifetime, men didn't admit to being as sensitive as women to physical imperfections. But most importantly, as he told one of his children later in life, the "ray of light would be extinguished" if his eye were removed.

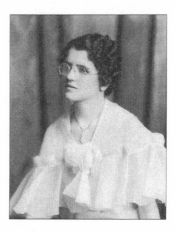

Jane Small, High School Senior Portrait, 1934

Sunday afternoon

Dear Irma,

A more appropriate time to write to that beloved
sister of mine I could never find. Anne is taking her usual
long nap, and Mario is in Indianapolis handeling a meeting
which concerns our old shhool Alumni. Incidently, they are
letting us have a meeting this spring.

I received both your letters this week--the hospital
forwarded the braille one so your efforts were not for nothing.
In fact, I enjoyed it very much, and I could read every word,
too. Your other letter came yesterday. Thanks for both of
them. Just keep it up and maybe I'll improve on my sorres-
pondence, too. I think about you often, but don't always
feel like writing.

Now that this operation is over I believe I am going to
have better health than ever before. I didn8t realize what
a constant burden that large eye was. The doctor said I would
be much better off now. If you are worrying about me --
please don't. I didn't suffer one bit. There was no pain
whatsoever. In fact, this was easier and more pleasant than
having my tonsils out. They didn't give me eather--just
a shot of something in the vein in my right arm put me to
sleep, and I felt nothing until I awakened hours later. It
was so simple and I had no shock at all, so I really had a
fine time at the hospital. The food was very good and there
was plenty. I had nice roomates, and the nurses were as
sweet as any I ever have met.

I came home last Sunday and for a few days I took it
easy, but I am back on the job again.

Pop and Elvie camned last Tuesday evening, and said
they would come down soon and bring you along. I couldn't
get them to say just when, it seems to depend on the weather.

I had a card from Ruth while I was in Indianapolis. She
said Paul had run into a tree and their car was in the garrage
again and that no one was hurt.

Yesterday I went back to Indianapolis to a checkup.
The eye has healed olokay, so that I can go to Chicago any
time. We are writing tomorrow for an appointment. If they
will okay it we will go probably this Friday and have the
fitting done Saturday morning. If that time isn't available
We will try to get in on Monday morning.

If the folks should decide to come down be sure to have
them call first.

Must close now and get busy.

                              Write soon,

                                   With love,

                                        Jane

MARIO'S CAREER

CHARLES, MARIO'S ADORED older brother, had been elected City Court Judge in 1943. Nearing the end of his term, he decided that his law practice was so busy that he would not run for re-election.

Spurred by the vacancy, Mario reasoned that if Charles could be city judge, he could be a city judge too. It was a part-time position in the morning, enabling him to practice law in the afternoon. The idea of a steady income was appealing, and Mario hoped that the publicity from the campaign would help his law practice, as it had helped Charles. Mario was untested in politics but hoped that having the same last name would help him win a few votes. It was an easy decision to enter the 1947 race, though it proved to be a challenging year for Mario. He was now responsible for Jane and two children under five years old. He constantly worried about having enough money to pay the bills, and now he would have to pay for a campaign. Mario was extremely careful about paying for his own campaign expenses and did not want to be beholden to any special interest group or person. Keeping his integrity and reputation for his honest legal practice was of paramount importance to him.

MARIO PIERONI
DEMOCRAT FOR
JUDGE OF CITY COURT

● Your City Court Judge must hear a great variety of cases.

● An understanding of human nature and a sympathetic approach to human problems as well as a basic knowledge of the law are essential.

● If you believe that I possess these qualifications, I would welcome and greatly appreciate your vote next Tuesday.

MY NUMBER ON THE VOTING MACHINE IS C-10. THANK YOU.

The Star Press, Muncie, Indiana
May 04, 1947

Running for election meant that he attended innumerable Democratic party bean suppers and meetings, keeping him from spending evenings with his family. He had been a popular speaker since beginning his law practice and rarely turned down an invitation to speak to Boy Scouts, church groups, or civic clubs. He was comfortable talking about his Seeing Eye dog and how he managed as a blind person, but he knew that the public would question how a blind person could be a judge. Through innumerable meetings, talks, interviews, and occasional newspaper advertisements, he worked hard to gain the voters' confidence.

Mario anxiously awaited the returns on election night downtown at the Democratic Party headquarters. His fears turned to elation as the vote showed that he'd not only beat his opponent but had garnered more votes than anyone on either side of the ballot. With a new confidence, he began planning his fall campaign. He needed to convince not only his opponent's supporters, but also Republicans to vote for him.

About a month after the primary election, Mario was at home and decided that it was time to take Carla out for a walk. He went upstairs, calling her name. She didn't respond, surprising Mario. Normally she'd be excitedly moving about, thumping her tail against the doorway or wall to greet him. His foot bumped into her; he reached down and discovered that Carla was dead on the floor next to his bed. Mario was shocked. The eight-year-old dog had not shown any signs of being ill.

Heartbroken at the loss of his trusted companion of seven years, the following morning Mario called the Seeing Eye and reported the sad news. Having found life-changing freedom with Carla, he knew that he needed to get another dog. He signed up for the next class. While the classes were free, he lost the income from his practice for three weeks and had to pay for his traveling expenses. He felt bad about leaving Jane alone with Anne and baby John but was comforted that his parents and Charles lived close by in case she needed help.

Still grieving Carla, Mario traveled alone by train to Morristown, New Jersey. He was soon matched with a large German shepherd named Baron. Although he was experienced working with a dog, Baron was much younger than Carla and had his own personality. The training took about three weeks, as Mario and Baron had much to learn about each other and needed to develop a bond between them. Once the instructors were convinced that they were a safe team, Mario and Baron were cleared to go home. They arrived back in Muncie in mid-July 1947, and Mario began planning his fall election campaign.

His intelligence and integrity, along with the numerous speeches, newspaper articles, and advertisements proclaiming his capabilities helped propel Mario to victory. Having a popular brother as the former city court judge also helped his campaign. Since they had the same last name, Mario laughingly said, "People didn't vote for me, they voted for my brother." Mario received the second highest number of votes on the Democratic ticket and was sworn into office on January 1, 1948. He was thirty-three years old.

Mario knew he had a lot to prove, not only as a young judge but as a blind one. Many people openly wondered how he could be a judge if he couldn't see. Mario used his Braille typewriter to take notes and had a bailiff to maintain order. Since he couldn't see a defendant's facial expressions, he devised alternative ways to get cues. He usually didn't have jury cases, so he kept the witness chair facing him, close to the bench. He created two questions to assess the defendant's honesty: Did what the accused have to say make sense? What was his physical reaction? Mario knew that if a person had nothing to hide, he would generally open his mouth and speak clearly. A dishonest defendant usually wouldn't look directly at the judge, instead turning his head away or looking down. Mario could tell by the way the accused's voice projected which way he was looking.

He also kept the witness chair in need of oil. If the questions embarrassed the person or he wasn't telling the truth, he often began squirming, which caused the chair to squeak. The amount of squeaking correlated with the defendant's discomfort and cued the judge to consider that the defendant may be lying. Mario was aware that there was no definitive way to know if a person was lying, so he usually found other evidence or witnesses that helped him to make a final judgment.

The inmates at the jail spread a rumor that a person could figure out which way Judge Pieroni would rule by watching Baron's tail. If his tail swished back and forth, supposedly the judge would find you guilty. There was no truth to that, of course, but Mario laughed at the jailhouse story.

He handled a variety of cases in court, including intoxicated driving, traffic violations, domestic violence, assault and battery, and other minor offenses. He assessed fines and didn't hesitate to send someone to jail if he thought they deserved it. The newspapers covered his decisions daily; people were curious how he would do as the first blind judge in Muncie.

Although news coverage of his decisions was favorable and his colleagues seemed to approve of his work, he knew that his every move was on display, both in and out of the courtroom. The only place that he could relax was at home, out of the public eye.

•• •
: •:

NOT A MATCH

PREOCCUPIED WITH HIS career and community activities, Mario didn't notice that Baron was becoming very attached to baby John. Every evening, Jane secured John in his highchair and gave him small pieces of meat and vegetables for dinner. Baron sat next to him, ready for the boy to start their game. John took a bite of meat and held it over the side of his highchair. Baron very carefully took it out of his fingers, never touching or biting him. John smiled but didn't laugh; neither dog nor boy made a sound. They were so quiet that Mario wasn't aware of the game until one evening when he left Baron's metal collar and dog tags on. He heard it rattle as Baron took a bit of meat from John's outstretched hand, triggering a suspicion that the dog was doing something forbidden. That ended their food game. Mario decided not to allow Baron into the kitchen during meals, because The Seeing Eye had emphasized never to feed the dog at the table. Dogs are notorious for begging, and The Seeing Eye did not want their dogs to be ill-behaved at home or in public.

Mario soon became aware that when John was sleeping, Baron would go over and lie by the crib, guarding him. As John toddled around the house, Baron followed him. While Mario was aware that

Baron seemed very attached to John, it never occurred to him that a problem could be developing with the dog.

One late summer day, two of the older neighborhood girls, Shirley and Mary Ellen, were playing with Anne and John on the step by the front sidewalk. Baron and Mario went out to make sure that they weren't too close to the street. Just as they were approaching, Mary Ellen picked up the toddler and handed him to Shirley.

Baron lunged at Shirley, who screamed, "Ow! He bit me!"

Mario instinctively jerked Baron's leash and held him back. "What? Baron bit you? Where did he get you?"

"He bit my ear. And it's bleeding!" cried Shirley.

"I'm so sorry! I can't believe that Baron bit you. Anne, help me bring John inside. I'll tie Baron down and come right back out. I'll bring you a clean washcloth for your ear."

Shaken, Mario and the children climbed the porch steps.

"Mom! Baron bit Shirley!" Anne loudly announced upon entering the living room.

"What? Oh no!" Jane came hurriedly from the kitchen. "Is she bleeding?"

"Yes, but I don't think that her ear will fall off. That's where he bit her," said Anne.

"Anne, watch John while I get something to stop the bleeding. Mario, how could this happen?"

"I don't know! I can't imagine him biting a child. This is awful. I need to get back outside," said Mario as he finished tying Baron's leash to the eyelet screwed into the wall.

Hearing the commotion, Shirley's parents had crossed the street and were assessing the injury when Mario returned to the scene.

"It's okay, Mario. She'll be just fine. It drew a little blood, but it's already stopped bleeding," said her father, Ray.

"I'm so sorry. I'm just stunned. I can't believe that he bit Shirley. Why would he do that?"

"Maybe Baron didn't like me holding John," said Shirley. "He bit me just as Mary Ellen gave him to me."

"Baron loves John, but I can't imagine him biting you just for holding him. This is very serious. I'll have to call the Seeing Eye tomorrow. I'm sorry, Mary Ellen. I hope that your ear is going to be all right."

"She'll be fine, Mario. We'll see you later," said Ray.

The next morning, Mario called The Seeing Eye and reported the incident. "You'll have to bring him back. Baron would be okay with somebody that didn't have any children, but you have a problem. Things have gone too far. When can you get to Morristown?"

For the second time within a year, Mario was forced to leave his work and family suddenly. He rescheduled court cases and found a temporary replacement judge. Losing the income from his law practice worried him, but he had no choice. He needed another dog. Once again, he said goodbye to Jane and the children and boarded the train for the long trip back to Morristown.

The thought of saying goodbye to a dog that he'd grown fond of was painful. Mario decided to lessen the sting by getting off the train early, in New York City, for a last "fling" together before returning to Morristown. On a bright early fall morning, they left Grand Central Station and walked down Fifth Avenue. He decided to get a little gift for Jane and went into a store. He had no idea which store he'd wandered into, although he could tell by the cool air and hushed atmosphere that it was likely a store with expensive items.

A clerk approached him and asked in icy tones, "May I help you?" "Yes, can you tell me the name of this store?"

"Sir, you are in Tiffany's."

Mario knew that he could not afford to buy anything at Tiffany's, but he wanted to save face, so he asked, "Which floor has the figurines?" He figured that he might be able to afford a little one.

"They are on the third floor. Go straight back to the elevators and someone will help you."

The elevator doors closed behind them as Mario hesitated on the third floor, wondering which way he should go and hoping that Baron's tail wouldn't knock a pricey porcelain figure to the floor.

"Sir, how may I help you?" asked another clerk, who eyed them suspiciously.

"Yes, I'm looking for a small figurine for my wife."

"Right this way, sir." The clerk took Mario's arm and steered them around the displays of expensive and fragile items. "I have a lovely China statue of a woman with a parasol. It's only $75."

"Do you have anything cheaper than that?"

"Our cheapest figurine is $29. But sir, it's not nearly as attractive as the lady with the parasol."

Mario knew that he couldn't afford to spend that much (approximately $335, adjusted for inflation) on a useless dust catcher. He thanked the clerk for his time and left, rather embarrassed at having wandered into such an exclusive store where he and Baron clearly didn't belong.

A little farther down the block, he tried again. This time he found a candy store, where he bought a box of chocolates for Jane. Back out in the sunshine on the crowded sidewalks of Fifth Avenue, he continued his walk until it was time to return to the train station and his final train ride with Baron.

For the third time at The Seeing Eye, he anxiously awaited meeting his new companion.

The handler finally brought an energetic young German Shepherd, named Uno, who happily licked his new master's hand. The Seeing Eye named each litter by the alphabet, so he was in the 'U' litter. Mario wondered how they could come up with many names starting with 'U' but accepted the name "Uno" and began training. The duo worked well together and completed the training in only two weeks.

Uno and Mario arrived in Muncie in early October 1948. Uno adjusted well to his new home, and Mario was glad to be bonding with a dog that wasn't distracted by children. Since he'd only had Baron for about eighteen months, he didn't consider the dog to have been a match and didn't count him as one of his dogs. Including Baron, Mario owned eight seeing eye dogs, although he always said that he'd had only seven in his lifetime. Apparently, The Seeing Eye agreed with Mario. The school gave him a trophy with a sculpture of a German Shepherd and a plaque that read:

The Seeing Eye celebrates with pride Mario Pieroni and his 59 years of loving and working with seven Seeing Eye dogs. Presented June 1, 2001.

• • •

HELPING OTHERS

BESIDES HIS DUTIES as Judge of City Court, practic-
ing law in the law firm of Pieroni & Pieroni, and raising a family,
Mario was very active in helping handicapped children. He was
a founder of the Delaware County Chapter of the Indiana Society
for Crippled Children and served in several capacities, including
president in 1945. The organization sold Easter Seals to raise money
to provide services such as education for the homebound (disabled
children usually didn't go to school) and money for medical care.
They also provided crutches, braces, hearing aids, and wheelchairs
to children. Fundraising letters with sheets of 100 colorful seals were
mailed to residents around Easter; recipients were encouraged to
send back a donation and use the seals to close envelopes, thereby
raising awareness of the plight of crippled children. Mario was chair
of both the local and state Easter Seals campaigns and helped to raise
thousands of dollars.

In 1945, the money raised by the Easter Seals campaign was
used to open a special school for handicapped children, the Harry
Mock School. Eleven children with various disabilities were the
first students taught in the well-equipped, cheerful basement of
Jefferson Elementary.

Without the leadership of the Society, those children would not have had any formal education. Local schools were not accessible to handicapped children, and those teachers did not have the expertise to work with them. The children were forced to stay home, isolated and illiterate. If not for the Indiana School for the Blind, Mario would have been one of those children.

But Mario wanted to do more than just raise money for the school. Once a week, he went on his lunch hour to teach Braille and offer encouragement to two visually impaired students. To celebrate Thanksgiving 1946, the local morning paper, *The Muncie Star,* sent a photographer to document the annual turkey luncheon at the school. Under the title, "Thankful, Though Blind," the picture depicts Mario and Carla standing next to a young blind boy with his lunch tray in the school cafeteria. Mario has his hand on the boy's shoulder; the caption quotes Mario as saying to the boy that handicapped persons, though unable to do some of the things their friends can accomplish, still have a great many things to be thankful for on this Thanksgiving Day. He added that "a handicapped person should be thankful for the facilities of which he still has control, and by using them to the best of his ability, and with the able assistance of his instructors, he can convert his handicap to an asset which he may use to serve himself and his community."

The Muncie Junior Chamber of Commerce recognized Mario for his community service by awarding him the prestigious "Outstanding Young Man of 1948" in a ceremony at the Masonic Temple auditorium. An editorial appearing the next day in the Muncie Evening Press noted that when he was called to the speaker's platform, "Mario Pieroni stood straight and strong before some five hundred men who had risen to their feet in silent tribute...Tears came to the blinded eyes and Judge Mario

Pieroni could not have been living in darkness at that moment…He had heard… that of all the fine young men considered, Judge Pieroni had been the unanimous choice of the committee." The editorial then stated that "it must have been the happiest moment in Judge Pieroni's life and his only regret was that 'my good wife' wasn't there to share this honor with him." His prizes included a pin, a certificate, and a tobacco humidor. He accepted them graciously, but since he never smoked tobacco, he brought it home and laughingly gave it to Jane.

The Eastern Indiana Notre Dame Club honored him as "Notre Dame Man of the Year 1949." The club presented him with a scroll recognizing "his life and example, his devotion to family, his interest in civic affairs, his Catholic action, [which] proved him to be a Notre Dame man in the rich significances of moral, responsible leadership for which his Notre Dame training equipped him." Mario is beaming in the newspaper picture, standing next to a man holding the scroll that he would never be able to see.

Believing that mental well-being was just as important as physical health, Mario didn't hesitate when asked to join with a group of citizens to form the Delaware County chapter of the Indiana Mental Hygiene Society. The group was front page news of *The Muncie Star* in January 1949, complete with a photo of the committee members, including Mario and his dog, Uno. The society worked to bring about public knowledge of mental illness, its causes, and treatment, with the goal of breaking through the stigma often associated with mental illness. Only two years later, the group opened the Child Guidance Center in Muncie to provide counseling for families and children.

Although he often saw the worst in people, he still maintained hope for a better world. Mario was president of the Muncie chapter of Optimist International in 1950. According to their website, the service group is dedicated to "providing hope and positive vision. Optimists bring out the best in youth, our communities and ourselves." Exhorting local members to "give of their time and efforts to make this a better world in which to live," Mario spent hours traveling and speaking to Optimist chapters around Indiana, giving speeches about his life. Newspaper articles detailing his speeches rarely mentioned how he traveled to those speaking engagements, but the *Terre Haute Tribune* photographer was at the train station when Jane, Mario, and Uno arrived on December 6, 1953, when their fourth child was just four months old. It must have been a special occasion for Jane to leave her children for a day trip to Terre Haute, since she rarely accompanied Mario to his civic talks.

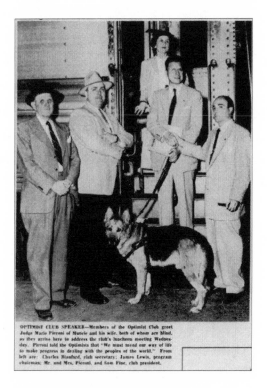

OPTIMIST CLUB SPEAKER—Members of the Optimist Club greet Judge Mario Pieroni of Muncie and his wife, both of whom are blind, as they arrive here to address the club's luncheon meeting Wednesday. Pieroni told the Optimists that "We must mend our way of life to make progress in dealing with the peoples of the world." From left are: Charles Blanford, club secretary; James Lewis, program chairman; Mr. and Mrs. Pieroni, and Sam Fine, club president.

The Terre Haute Tribune
December 6, 1953

Jane was also a member of the Opti-Mrs. Club, the women's version of Optimist International, and served in several leadership capacities, including president in 1959. Naturally a quiet person who usually preferred staying in the background at most social events, Jane ably led business meetings and introduced the monthly speakers. But one of her duties was to host the annual membership tea, and the *Muncie Evening Press* was there to take a photo of Jane and three other ladies who were gathered around the white tablecloth-covered table laden with a punch bowl, flowers, and cookies. Jane is the only one not smiling in the photo. It must have been stressful for her to host the membership tea at her home; she constantly worried about the house being clean and neat, knowing that visitors would be very curious to see the inside of a blind woman's home.

Jane was also featured as speaker at meetings for three organizations: The Newcomers Club, the sorority Delta Theta Tau, and the Burris Mothers' Club. The articles announcing Jane as speaker focused on naming those in attendance and describing the decorations. No information was given about Jane's subject matter, but presumably her topics included her experiences as a blind wife and mother.

• •
•
•

RITA ARRIVES AND MARIO IS DRAFTED

HOLDING THE SCREAMING baby—her third child— firmly to her chest, Jane maneuvered her way from the changing table to the crib. She hated the cluttered bedroom, which had been too small even for Anne and John. In addition to their twin beds, she'd barely managed to cram a changing table and crib into the space, leaving very little room for walking. If she tripped over a toy or lost her balance, Jane worried that her newborn, Rita Jane, would slip from her grip and fall.

Sweat dripped from her face onto the baby's shoulder. Every window was open, but with no breeze, the unrelenting late July, 1950 heat made the cramped bedroom feel even smaller. Rita whimpered as Jane bent over the crib, feeling the sheet for the right spot to lay her precious bundle. Rita quieted, and Jane exhaled a sigh of relief. She hoped that the baby could sleep in the hot room. As she turned on a small table fan, she heard three-year-old John arguing with Anne in the living room. He needed his nap, but she was afraid that he'd wake up the baby. With only two bedrooms, juggling the needs of three young children was stressful. She decided to put John into her bed and laid down with him to help him sleep.

When Jane and John awoke from their naps, Mario was home and listening to Anne read a book. Still groggy and tired from the heat, Jane was not in a good mood.

"Mario! We have to do something. I can't stand it anymore. We don't have room for three children in this house," Jane said as she leaned against the archway to the living room. Anne stopped reading and looked at each parent, not wanting to get involved in an impending argument.

"Anne, thanks for reading to me. Why don't you go outside and get some fresh air?" Relieved, Anne put down the book and skipped out of the living room.

Turning to his wife, Mario said, "Now Jane, it won't be much longer. My Dad just can't throw those renters out of the house. We'll have to be patient. Mr. Johnson will move out as soon as his wife dies. Then we'll have plenty of space."

"Your father is too nice. And why can't that old lady just die? She's had cancer forever. I'm tired of waiting. We need those three bedrooms. Anne and the baby can share a room, and John will have his own. It will make bedtime so much easier. And it's not safe now. That little room is so full of furniture that I can hardly walk in there. I'm afraid that I'll trip and drop Rita."

"I know. I feel sorry for you, and I'm sorry for poor Mrs. Johnson."

"They've lived two doors down on the other side of your parents' house for three years, and they've never been friendly. I don't feel that sorry for her. I'd hoped that we could be in our new house before Rita was born. There's a lot of painting and wallpapering that needs to be done. Now we'll have to stay in here until that work is finished. I just can't have three kids in the house while they're painting."

"No, we can't live there while they're painting. But we're okay here for now. At least we have a roof over our heads."

"It may be fine for you. You aren't here twenty-four hours a day in the heat, trying to cook and clean and change diapers. And not knowing when we can move makes it even harder. I can't even get the painters lined up."

"Now, Jane. You shouldn't wish that poor woman to die any faster. We just have to be patient."

"Well, I can't wait for that extra half bath and the third bedroom. All the rooms are so much bigger than what we have now. I'm going to need an interior designer to help me with colors. Anne is too young to help, and I don't want your mother's opinion. At least I can decide on paint colors and start thinking about where to put the furniture."

When the unfortunate neighbor passed away in late August 1950, Jane happily began planning the move. With help from the designer, Jane decided on a medium shade of green paint for the living and dining rooms. Wall-to-wall carpet was *de rigueur* in the 1950s. Mario and Jane liked it because it absorbed sound, thus reducing annoying echoes. Area rugs were dangerous, and Jane didn't want to worry about tripping over them, so she had carpet everywhere but the kitchen, breakfast room, and bathrooms. Ever practical, Jane chose a beige carpet. It went with the furniture and wouldn't show dog hair.

The renovations were finished in October. Jane hired movers to carry the furniture and boxes the short distance two houses away. Eletta watched the children while Antonio directed the furniture placement. Even Anne helped by carrying her toys to her new room.

Jane loved their new house; the extra bathroom saved steps and arguments, and John, now almost four years old, was happy to have his own bedroom. Anne shared a room with baby Rita, but she but didn't mind sharing. Her new room was larger, and she liked having space for her books.

Jane worked hard to decide where to put every item in the house. She was a firm believer in "a place for everything and everything in its place." If she wanted something, she needed to know where to find it. If it wasn't put back in its proper place, it was much more difficult for her to find. She couldn't just look at a shelf and pick up an item. If it wasn't there, she had to use her hands to feel around, often just missing what she was looking for. Surprisingly, Jane was so good   at remembering where she placed things that she rarely wasted time trying to find something. "Put it back where you found it" was repeated often in the household, and even Mario didn't dare to disobey the rule.

While Jane was busy with the children and settling into the house, Mario continued to practice law and entered his third year as city judge. He became even more active in the Democratic Party and was drafted to run for mayor in the May 1951 primary. He'd planned on running for reelection for judge, but party leaders were concerned with corruption in the incumbent Democrat mayor's office. They convinced Mario, with his honest and good reputation, that he would be the perfect candidate. Prominent Muncie leaders joined in, assuring him that they would donate money and time to his campaign. Flattered, Mario bowed to their pressure. Without consulting Jane, and just eight months after the birth of their third child, Mario decided that running for mayor would be his opportunity to rid the city of corruption.

Jane was furious about his unilateral decision. How dare he make such an important commitment without her! She remembered the many nights when he was out making speeches or attending rubber chicken dinners campaigning for judge in 1947. Now she had three young children, including Rita—who, as a toddler, required constant attention. She had to focus and be mindful of what the children were doing at every moment. She couldn't visually see a misdeed and correct the child. She had to stop what she was doing, walk over, find the child, check their hands, and feel around the area to investigate what they were doing. Anne helped with the younger children, but she was in school weekdays. Raising three children and doing all the household chores without help was exhausting. She needed Mario home at night, but all too often, he was campaigning for an office that she didn't want him to win.

Jane dreaded the thought of going to endless political dinners and ceremonies. Aside from the difficulty of having a suitable wardrobe and arranging transportation to events, she found it hard to chat in a noisy environment. She couldn't catch someone's eye to initiate conversation. She worried about being stuck on a chair, alone and isolated in a room full of laughing people. Jane couldn't move around an unfamiliar room by herself; she was dependent upon someone else to walk with her. If she needed to use the restroom, it was embarrassing to have to locate and ask another woman to accompany her there. Social functions were stressful, and she'd much prefer to be home with the children.

As the campaign progressed, it became apparent that some people did not want the mayor's office to be cleaned up. Jane became concerned for Mario's safety, especially after an anonymous phone threat. The caller said that they knew that he walked home every day and where he lived. Jane was frightened. What would she do if something happened to Mario? How could she raise three children alone, without any way to make a living for herself?

Mario was less concerned about his own personal safety. He thought that the caller just wanted him out of the race and wouldn't follow through. He continued his campaign, giving frequent radio talks and attending events.

His work earned him a May primary victory, beating the incumbent mayor by a three-to- one margin. He stepped up the pace for the fall election but couldn't heal the scars from the primary. He was soundly beaten in a GOP landslide that year, as almost every Republican on the ballot was elected to local offices. Disappointed by the loss, he concentrated on his law practice, which had grown to include three partners, and did not pursue another public office for twenty years.

Jane was quite relieved at the outcome, although it was difficult for her to comfort her husband. She couldn't change the results, nor did she wish that it had been different. She assumed that Mario would be home more in the evenings, but instead of politicking, he resumed his old habit of walking next door after dinner to visit his parents. Jane's relief quickly turned into irritation as once again she was abandoned at night to manage the children.

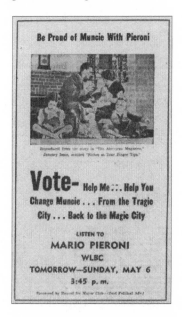

Muncie Evening Press,
May 5, 1951

•• ••

1953: A VERY GOOD YEAR

"JANE IS PREGNANT again? What does she want another one for?" Ruth held the telephone receiver tightly to her ear, anxious to hear more news about her sister's pregnancy.

"I have no idea," replied Irma, the oldest of the three sisters. "I don't know how she manages the three children that she has now. I only have two kids and they're a handful."

"When is she due?"

"She told me sometime in the middle of August."

"Ugh! You know that my Paula Kay's birthday is in August. I know how hot and miserable it is to be fat in the summer. Does Pop know about Jane?" asked Ruth.

"Yes. He's worried about them managing such a big family and how Mario can afford to feed a family of six. But Mario's a lawyer, and I'll bet that he makes enough money. I told Pop that they'll be fine. Jane is a good mother and she'll be able to handle four kids, but I don't envy her having a baby at age forty. That wears me out just thinking of it," said Irma.

"Me, too. Thanks for calling. I need to start dinner now. Bye," said Ruth as she hung up the phone.

Irma and Ruth weren't alone in wondering how Jane could manage four children.

Reaction was muted on Mario's side as well, although Eletta and Antonio looked forward to the new addition. Neighbors and friends gossiped among themselves about the pregnancy, speculating on how a blind woman could raise one child, much less four.

Four children would be costly, and Mario worried about making ends meet. It would be humiliating to fail as a lawyer and be forced to borrow money from his parents or brother. While his law practice was growing, Mario's income was unpredictable. Some years were better than others.

Having no car or other large expenses, the family lived simply and within their means. They had one telephone and one television for the children. They rarely ate at restaurants and didn't travel on vacations. Mario hoped that his fourth child would be healthy and the necessary additional expenses low.

Jane's main luxury was a cleaning woman who came once a week to help with the heavy cleaning. She mopped the floors, vacuumed, and cleaned the bathrooms. It would have taken Jane a long time to mop the kitchen floor, and even then, she couldn't see if she'd missed any spots. The children weren't supposed to leave toys on the floor, but if a crayon had fallen off a table, Jane didn't want to ruin the vacuum by running over it. Mario's guide dog shed constantly. Despite Jane's best efforts, it was impossible for her to sweep up all of it. She couldn't see or hear the fur fly away from her broom and dustpan. The cleaning woman saved Jane much time and worry, giving her the satisfaction that at least once a week, her house was thoroughly clean.

With no income of her own, Jane was completely financially dependent upon Mario. She couldn't see to write a check, so Jane had no checking account. Credit cards were ten years in the future. Mario gave her a weekly cash allowance for groceries. She spent it very carefully and usually had some money left over. She kept the extra cash in a box in a dresser drawer and used it for special things that she wanted but didn't want to ask Mario to buy. If she needed to purchase something, he didn't refuse her request, but at times they disagreed on what was necessary for the children. Jane was determined that the children would have nice clothes, plenty of toys, and bikes to ride. Mario often questioned her purchases, but he usually relented. He mostly wanted assurance that Jane was spending his earnings wisely.

In the 1960s when the main department store downtown, Ball Stores, introduced credit cards, Jane experienced a new freedom. She didn't have to ask Mario up front for cash to buy clothes or makeup. She simply took out the little plastic card and it was paid for! They developed a routine when she returned home with Mario asking, "Did you have a successful shopping trip?"

Jane always answered, "Oh yes! It was a lot of fun and I got what I needed." She didn't see any reason to give details. He didn't really care about the dress that she'd bought. When the bill came due, Mario's secretary wrote the check. He didn't complain, so Jane assumed that she wasn't buying too much. She didn't like being dependent on him for all her money, but she had no choice. She was a housewife, and there was no way that she could ever earn any money on her own.

* * *

The summer of 1953 was miserably hot, with no escape from the heat. An occasional light breeze blew through the open windows but did little to cool the house. Jane was eight months pregnant and exhausted, worn down by the constant high temperatures and household chores. Her belly made it difficult to do almost anything, and her hands and feet were swollen. After Rita was born, the doctor had insisted that she stay a week in the hospital, not for any medical complications, but to allow her time to rest and recover. She didn't mind having her meals brought to her and sleeping as much as she needed. She hoped that her doctor would again order her to stay for a week after this pending birth.

The only time she could relax was when three-year-old Rita took a nap. Rita was an active child who required constant supervision, more so than the first two children. Anne kept an eye on her at times, but Jane didn't want to burden her ten-year-old daughter. It wasn't her job to be a full-time babysitter, although it was helpful when she told her mother that Rita was getting into trouble. Yet Rita's mischievous escapades often escaped detection. One of her favorite activities was to tie miniscule knots in the cords that pulled open the draperies. Jane discovered her handiwork when she tried to close the draperies in the evenings; the knots were almost impossible to get out. Jane hoped that her next baby would be less active.

PART TWO

• • • •
•

ABANDONED

I'M MARY, THE youngest child of Mario and Jane. The previous chapters, written in third person, were based upon stories my parents told and were captured on both audio and video tapes. Transcriptions of those interviews and reminisces enabled me to quote them accurately, since I wasn't there during that time. I didn't arrive in the world until 1953, but the tapes, combined with years of hearing their stories and extensive research, helped me to imagine their lives.

Mom told me that she went into labor on the evening of August 12. Dad took my siblings next door to our grandparents, and his Uncle Joe drove them to the hospital. Mom's labor was uneventful, and I, their fourth child, was born the next morning and named Mary Teresa. As anticipated, Mom's doctor insisted that she stay in the hospital for a week of rest. He knew that as soon as she was home, she'd be up and working. He wanted her to feel rested before allowing her to leave the hospital. And he was right. Mom was grateful that she had the extra rest, as there was little time to recover when she got home.

My arrival necessitated some changes with bedroom assignments. There were only three bedrooms upstairs. Rita and Anne shared a room, while John had his own. There wasn't enough space for me in the girls' room and my parents didn't want to put a crib in John's room. A year before my birth, an addition had been built to the first floor, just off the dining room toward the back of the house. It was used as a den and ironing room. Mom liked to iron there because she could keep the wooden ironing board set up. She always put away the iron but felt that taking the heavy board down wasted her energy. It was quiet there, but still close enough to the living room where the children played. She could listen for any fighting or trouble and still get the ironing done.

Mom and Dad decided to move John downstairs to the addition. They bought bunk beds, removed the ironing board, and made it into a cozy bedroom. John, who wasn't quite seven years old, was upset by the move. He didn't like being so far away from the rest of the family. Mom didn't realize that he felt rejected or abandoned until he complained as an adult, and while she wished that there had been another bedroom upstairs, they unfortunately didn't have any better options.

Although John felt isolated, his room wasn't far from the living room, where the new black-and-white television was installed in the corner by the fireplace. My siblings loved to watch television, especially *Raymer of the Jungle* and *Howdy Doody*. Rita, John, and Anne sat cross-legged on the floor, staring at the screen for as long as Mom would allow.

Mom set up my playpen in the dining room and often put me there while she did chores.

But I could see my siblings watching TV in the next room and wasn't happy about being stuck away from the action. My protesting cries made it impossible to hear the show, so Anne often rescued me, holding me in her lap. Of course, I stopped crying and happily watched the images flickering across the screen.

One warm fall afternoon, when I was three months old, Mom put me down for a nap in my blue baby carriage. I was told that I fussed briefly, then slowly quieted. John, who was six and a half, peered into the carriage and smiled at me. He thought, *Maybe she'd like to go for a ride. That will help make her sleep.* John heard Mom working in the kitchen and decided that he'd help her by taking me out for a walk.

He managed to get the carriage out the front door and down the steps. John turned left and began pushing the carriage down the sidewalk alongside busy Jackson Street. By the time he got to the corner, John decided that he was tired and laid down to rest on Mrs. Wellinger's front lawn. After a few minutes John got up and skipped home, leaving me and the carriage behind.

Soon after, the telephone rang in the front hall.

"Mrs. Pieroni? This is Mrs. Wellinger from down the street," said the neighbor urgently.

"Yes, hello," Mom replied, wondering why she was calling her.

"I just looked out my window, and I saw Mary in her carriage out on my front sidewalk. She's by herself. I don't see anybody with her, and I don't know how in the world she got there!"

"WHAT? I don't understand. She's taking a nap in her carriage! I just put her there a while ago. She can't be out on the sidewalk." Still trying to comprehend the situation, Mom paused, her heart pounding and panic building.

"I tell you, she's there. Do you want me to bring her home?"

"No, thank you. Anne and I will be right there."

Mom hung up the phone. "Anne, come here. We need to get Mary. Did you take her on a walk?"

"No, Mom. I've been playing with Rita. Where is Mary?"

"Mrs. Wellinger says that she's on the sidewalk in front of her house. Hurry! Let's go!" Mom, who was not a runner, practically ran down the sidewalk while holding onto Anne's left elbow.

"I see the carriage, Mom. And Mrs. Wellinger is there, too," said Anne.

Mom told me later that I was still asleep when they reached me, with Mom heaving a sigh of relief that I was safe.

After exchanging greetings, Mom said to her neighbor, "I don't know how Mary got here! Anne and Rita were playing together. I can't imagine that John would take her by himself, but it must have been him," said Mom, still shocked that her baby had been abandoned along a busy street. "Thanks again, Mrs. Wellinger," said Mom as they turned to push the carriage back home.

She was mortified that she hadn't heard John take the carriage and prayed that nobody would call child welfare to say that she was an unfit mother. She worked hard every day to prove that her blindness didn't interfere with raising four children. But a six year old leaving a baby alone on a sidewalk made her feel like an inadequate and neglectful mother. What if Mrs. Wellinger hadn't called her and instead called child welfare or the police? They could have accused her of child abandonment and taken her children away—her worst nightmare.

Luckily, there was no investigation, but that was the end of John's unsupervised walks with me.

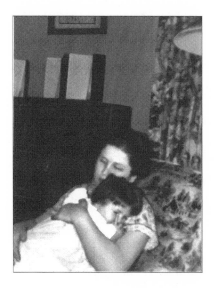

Jane and Mary

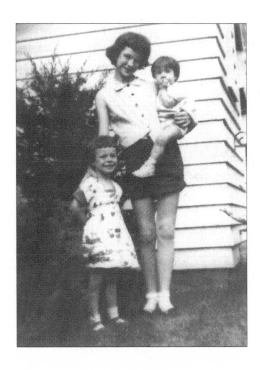

Rita, Anne, and Mary

••
•
•

MARY'S STORY

I GREW UP in a loving household with parents who were patient
and kind. Our family looked like other families who were at Sunday
Mass or on television (my main frame of reference as a child). Yet
Mom and Dad's eyes didn't light up when they saw me or darken
when I did something wrong. They had no idea what I looked like.
But that didn't matter. They saw me by touching my hair, counting
my toes, giving me a bath. They heard my voice break with tears when
I was upset and smiled when they heard laughter.

There was never a defining moment when I realized that my
parents were blind. An early clue for me was when, as a toddler,
I looked up into their eyes and saw nothing. No emotion, except for
the rare occasions when my father was angry. Then, his big, scary eye
got even bigger. His little eye, the one that had burst when he was
four, was permanently closed. He couldn't open that eye. His eyes
were frightening to me. My mother had artificial eyes. She could open
them, but those glass orbs closed the door to her soul.

Since I couldn't make eye contact with either of my parents,
I learned to listen to their voice tones instead of looking at their faces.
I didn't have to make eye contact to know that Mom was unhappy
that I'd stolen a cookie before dinner. As an adult, I've realized that

I have a difficult time making eye contact with anyone and must remind myself to look people in the eye. I'm more comfortable looking away while I listen to someone talk. It helps me to concentrate on what they're saying while I listen to their voice tone and hear the emotions underneath the words. I tend to get distracted if I try to watch a speaker's face.

Visual cues are harder for me to read. When I do try to gaze in someone's eyes, I have no idea what they're trying to tell me. I need auditory cues. The ubiquitous emojis on social media perplex me. I know the obvious smiley and unhappy faces, but I don't use the others because I'm not sure what they're trying to convey, and I'm afraid that I'll post something inappropriate.

But I heard the sound of love from my parents' voices and their gentle touches. My mother had a very tender touch as she gently brushed my hair, bathed my small body, and changed my cloth diapers. I was about five years old when I started walking as a guide with them instead of their holding my hand and watching for my safety. I still remember the feeling of their light grip on my elbow as we walked.

If I wanted to show my mother something—perhaps my doll—instead of holding it up for her visual inspection or approval, she instructed me to "put it in my hand and let me see it." She traced the outline of the doll's body with her fingers and felt the face, exclaiming what a pretty doll she was. I watched with great satisfaction as Mom examined my doll, then smiled as she handed it back, admonishing me to "take good care of your dolly."

In elementary school, my sister Rita and oldest sister Anne took the bus downtown to Van's Dance Studio every Saturday. Rita learned tap, ballet, and tumbling, while Anne concentrated on ballet. Ever the conscientious student, Rita often practiced her routines at home. As Mom forbade tap shoes on the tile kitchen floor, Rita solved that problem by climbing up on a built-in wooden table along one wall of the basement. It was perfect for a stage, and Rita put on many "shows," insisting that both parents come to watch her tap dance and sing. They dutifully clapped and cheered, providing her with the attention that she craved.

Always practical, I didn't care about putting on a show since they couldn't see me anyway. And I had zero talent or interest in dancing; I much preferred riding my bicycle. It wasn't until my own daughter put on shows that I realized that I never said, "Watch me, Mommy! Look what I can do!" Maybe I just didn't care to perform—I was a quiet child and preferred to stay in the background. But I never craved their attention, and even as a young child, I knew that since they couldn't see me, their cheering felt empty.

I took piano lessons from the second grade through middle school. I enjoyed the lessons, but like many children, I didn't practice enough. Playing for myself was fun, but I got too nervous while playing for others. I'd get distracted, lose focus, and make mistakes. I hated performing in the recitals; I still remember my sweaty hands on the piano keys. The Muncie newspapers used to publish accounts of my teacher Mrs. Maier's student recitals, naming every child and what they played. I found one article that said, "Mario Pieroni will play a duet with his nine-year-old daughter, Mary." I have no memory of that recital, but now I wish that videos had been invented. I'd love to see and hear that piece! I remember only one time that Dad played the piano at home. I was shocked at how good he was and asked why he didn't play more. He said, "I can't play well enough to suit me." And he never played the piano again.

Music filled the house. During the day, Mom listened to the local radio station. It played what's now called "elevator music"— mostly background music with lots of soaring strings. The living room had a stereo record player inside a stylish wood cabinet. My father had an eclectic collection of vinyl 33 rpm records, including classical music, musicals such as Oklahoma, and jazz albums. All were labeled in Braille. He often stacked four records on the spindle. The arm automatically dropped a new record when one side was finished, so he could sit comfortably in the overstuffed rocking chair, read his Braille magazine, and not have to get up when the record was over.

Because they lived in a dark world, Mom and Dad were acutely aware of sound. They taught me to listen to the sound of a bird singing; Dad knew many birds by their song. I'm attuned to birdsong as well. I stop and listen with delight to a bird's melody. Once a friend was chattering about nothing while I tried to listen to a cardinal. She was completely oblivious to the beautiful song. I impatiently hushed her so that I could listen. She looked at me with surprise but at least stopped talking briefly. She was puzzled why a bird was more important than her, when she had important things to say. I apologized but thought to myself that human talk isn't nearly as uplifting as the song of a cardinal.

The absence of sound when the four of us were young usually meant that a child was doing something they shouldn't. When Mom realized that we were too quiet, she'd come to check on us. Crayons were kept in a drawer and only brought out when she or Anne could supervise us. The scissors were hidden until we got old enough to be trusted not to cut our hair or injure ourselves. Mom did everything that she could to ensure that we'd be safe.

When I was eight years old, it was almost time for dinner, and I was starving. Mom was frying hamburgers in the electric skillet, which made enough noise that I thought she wouldn't hear me if I climbed up on the kitchen counter to reach the cookie cabinet. Stealthily, I swung my leg up onto the counter, then pulled myself up and opened the cabinet. Grabbing a Fig Newton, I quickly stuffed it into my mouth and tried to quietly lower myself down to the floor.

"Mary! What are you doing? I hear you over there."

"Um, nothing," I answered while trying frantically to swallow the gooey cookie.

"You have something in your mouth, don't you? Did you get a cookie?"

"No, I don't!" I protested weakly, knowing full well that I was busted.

"You'll ruin your dinner. You know better than to eat a cookie before dinner. Shame on you! Now go set the table."

It was very hard to misbehave around my parents. They heard everything. I wasn't a saint, but along with my Catholic upbringing, I developed a strong conscience and became a "good girl."

Besides, how could I dare disobey my blind mother and father? I don't remember what I did to provoke my mother when I was four, but I have a vivid memory of running around the dining room table being chased by Mom, who was wielding the flyswatter. That was the usual discipline, to get tapped on the legs with the flyswatter. Suddenly, I felt terribly ashamed that I'd made my blind mother chase me and stopped running to await my punishment. I vowed not to ever make her chase me again.

Besides teaching me to listen, Mom and Dad commented on the smells at home or while riding in the car. I can still hear Dad say, "My, that smells good!" when he came into the kitchen. When we went for rides in the car after Anne turned sixteen, I loved going past the Colonial Bakery and the smell of Colonial bread baking. Sixty years later, I still remember the yeasty aroma.

Our 1958 Chevy had no air conditioning, of course, so the windows were down during the summer. While my short hair blew wildly about, I heard Dad take a deep breath and say, "We must be passing a farm. I smell that earthy cow manure!" It was especially pungent after a summer rain; I still appreciate the fresh Indiana country air when I return for visits.

The sense of touch was especially important to Mom. She used her fingers not only to read Braille, but to wash dishes and clean surfaces. She felt every inch of a plate, moving her fingers in search of a crumb or baked-on residue. Before we had a dishwasher, she did the dishes by hand. Each plate, piece of silverware, pot, and skillet was washed with a dishcloth, then thoroughly inspected by her sensitive fingers for anything left behind. "What's that?" she said to herself, picking at a particle stuck to a plate. "It feels sticky. Must be rice." Satisfied that she'd removed the offending bit of rice, she dipped the plate back into the soapy water and scrubbed again. It was a long process, especially for an impatient child helping to dry the dishes. When I complained about how long it took her, she responded, "How else can I know if it's clean?"

Before the invention of permanent press in the mid-1960s, Mom sat on a stool behind the ironing board and ironed every wrinkled cotton shirt and handkerchief. The hot iron sizzled with steam as she moved it slowly and methodically across the fabric, feeling with her fingers for missed wrinkles. Sometimes her fingers got too close to the steam, and she jerked her hand back, softly murmuring, "Ouch!" But she didn't complain and went back to her task after cooling the finger quickly in her mouth.

When I was seven, she asked if I'd like to learn how to iron handkerchiefs. She showed me how to sprinkle a little water on the fabric, then move the iron back and forth. I felt quite grown-up that she trusted me with the dangerous, hot iron. One day she left the room while I was finishing up the last of Dad's handkerchiefs. I got distracted by our cat and stopped moving the iron while I watched her play. Mom came hurriedly back, asking "What's that smell? Something's burning!" Fortunately, it was only scorched and didn't catch fire, but I learned why you don't leave a hot iron on one spot for very long.

Mom knew all our clothes by touch, remembering the color by the feel of the fabric and shape of the piece. She knew that the smooth dress with buttons on the front was my red dress. Her memory was as good as my dad's when it came to our clothes. She knew which blouse belonged to which sister and offered opinions on which top should go with a particular skirt.

Mom did all the laundry, including hanging clothes back up in our closets. She never asked us to help, although I'm sure that I put my own clothes back when I was older.

I was in high school during the late 1960s, which was the height of the miniskirt fad. Of course, I wanted to wear what everyone else was wearing, and bought skirts that came a few inches above the knee. Every morning before school, I had to submit to an inspection. Mom reached down and felt from my waist down to the bottom of the hem. "Mary, that's too short. I don't know how you can wear it that short, especially in the winter." I wasn't about to admit that the cold winter wind blew up under my skirt and chapped my legs. I had to be fashionable. The temporary discomfort of walking to school in 20-degree temperatures was the price I was willing to pay.

Mealtimes were special to my parents. Dinner was always served by 6:00 p.m., sometimes earlier if Dad had to attend an evening meeting. All six of us gathered nightly around the long, narrow table that barely fit in the breakfast room. Eating together gave us time to review our day, and Dad often told funny stories about courthouse events and people. Politics were an important topic, although as a child, I asked to be excused because that was "grown-up talk" and I'd long since finished my meal.

On weekends and holidays, when meals were more leisurely and relatives sometimes joined us in the dining room, Mom and Dad liked nothing better than to linger after a meal and talk. Dad enjoyed the intellectual discourse, and although Mom joined in, my guess is that she was happy to rest after working hard to prepare the meal. Relaxing over coffee helped to revive her prior to doing the dishes.

It wasn't just talk that was important at meals. Enjoying each bite became a sensory experience. Since they had no visual cues, they never said, "Yum, this looks good," but often commented on how something smelled or was particularly flavorful. They noted that the strawberries smelled fresh or if the bananas were over-ripe; Mom and Dad could easily tell by smell and touch. If how food looks is important in our expectations of how things will taste, then how the food smelled was the equivalent to Mom and Dad.

And yes, they fed themselves and cut their own meat. Mom used her fork to "feel around" on her plate to look for food. Peas were hard to keep on a fork, but she often mixed them with applesauce, making them easier to scoop up. As an adult, when they came to my house for dinner, I'd use a clock analogy and tell them that the meat was at twelve o'clock, the potatoes at three and the broccoli at nine o'clock. Knowing where everything was on the plate made it easier to decide where to begin eating.

Besides never leaving toys on the floor, Mom's other major rule was "no eating in the living room." We could only eat at the table, where spills could be easily wiped up and crumbs swept from the floor. Our black-and-white television was in the living room, and I have no memory of ever eating and watching TV. She was afraid that we'd make a mess in the living room and that someone would drop by and think that she was a poor housekeeper. She worried a lot about appearances.

We rarely ate out when I was growing up. It was too expensive for a family of six; eating out was reserved for very special occasions. Carryout was unusual in the 1950s and '60s and was something that those with cars enjoyed. Mom rarely got a break from cooking, but occasionally we'd eat lunch on a Saturday while shopping at the best department store in Muncie, Ball Stores. It had a cafeteria, and I read the menu and described the dishes to Mom. It was tricky to balance both of our trays while Mom held my elbow. If we were lucky, an employee would notice and carry her tray to our table.

I liked cafeterias. Mom often asked, "What looks good today?" as we began our slow walk down the line. Of course, everything looked good, especially the cakes and pies which were always displayed first. I tried to describe them as tantalizingly as possible, and often my ploy worked, as she suggested that we each get a piece.

In restaurants, it irritated me when the waitress held out a menu for Mom. Couldn't she tell that Mom was blind? Apparently not. Some waitresses would silently stare at her face, not understanding why she wasn't reaching for the menu. I often had to rescue the woman by saying, "We just need one menu, thanks." It didn't bother Mom that the waitress was standing there waiting for her to take the menu, but I was once again reminded that my Mom was different. And being different in any way was definitely not cool.

If Mom or Dad knew what they wanted to order, it was easy. I only had to look for the desired items on the menu and read it to them to confirm their order. Other times, they'd ask me to read the whole menu, which as I grew older, I found embarrassing and time-consuming.

It was embarrassing because who else reads the menu out loud? And I was hungry, too. I didn't want to spend ten minutes reading the menu. Sometimes I had to repeat the dish's description because they didn't remember it from the first reading. I learned which foods they didn't like, so I skipped over those items. Why read them something they won't order?

Reading the menus aloud set us apart, but even worse was the typical waitress who couldn't make eye contact with Mom or Dad, so she'd look at me and say, "What does she want?" as if they were deaf or too stupid to speak for themselves. It was demeaning to them. I learned as a six- or seven-year-old to ignore the question and say, "Mom, what would you like?" When I was a teenager, I'd retort, "I don't know. Why don't you ask her?" I understand that many people don't know what to say to a blind person, but it's not hard. Just treat them like anyone else!

$$\bullet \bullet \bullet\bullet$$
$$\bullet$$

FREEDOM

WHEN YOU WERE a child, did you ever close your eyes to see what it would be like to be blind? Perhaps you tried walking a few steps with your arms outstretched, hands waving as you tried to avoid walking into a wall. I couldn't keep my eyes closed for very long. It was too scary. I was greatly relieved when I opened my eyes and saw my familiar bedroom. I didn't want to be blind. That had to be the worst thing ever. But Mom and Dad didn't seem to be scared. They had already experienced the worst that could happen—losing their sight. Being blind was normal for them. I shuddered when I thought about losing my sight and prayed that it wouldn't happen to me.

Dad often said that it is easier to lose your sight when you're young and don't know what you're missing. He expressed sympathy for those who had vision, then lost it as an adult, saying that it's much harder to adjust to a dark world after always being able to see. Children adapt very quickly and concentrate more on what they can do rather than what they can't. Both of my parents were very fortunate to have understanding siblings and nurturing parents, which undoubtedly allowed them to flourish.

Neither of them felt sorry for themselves. They didn't waste time on self-pity. Both were practical-minded problem-solvers who saw their blindness as an obstacle to overcome, not something that prevented them from living. They weren't going to sit in a chair and be waited on. They wanted to live their lives independently and with dignity, making their own way in life.

Yet their blindness caused much frustration because it prevented them from doing many things that the sighted take for granted. Mom couldn't tell if her lipstick was on straight, and Dad didn't know if he'd spilled a spot of soup on his tie. Mirrors were useless to them; we children became their mirrors when Mom asked if her dress was clean.

I was glad that I could see and help them by reading the mail or the directions on a frozen pie. I didn't mind walking with Mom's hand on my elbow, guiding her safely down the sidewalk to the bus stop or church—at least not until I was an adolescent. Then I was embarrassed that people stared at us, and I felt constrained by her hand and having to be always on alert for hazards. I am sure that my siblings felt the same way, because we used to shake our heads and mouth "It's your turn!" while pointing at each other, waiting until one felt guilty enough to say verbally, "Mom, do you want to walk with me?" We didn't want her to know that we were fighting over who had to walk with her, so the negotiations were all done silently. I was the youngest, so I rarely won, but it was such a delicious feeling of freedom when Rita or John relented. I could skip or walk as fast as I wanted.

As an adult, Anne told me how free she had felt when she went away to college. She didn't care about freedom in the sense that many teenagers use the term. They usually mean that with no parents around, they can party all they want. Anne wasn't interested in partying. Her freedom was walking alone, without worrying about being responsible for a parent's safety. She was free to study and read all she wanted;

no more monitoring her younger siblings. Anne became accountable only to herself.

Having blind parents meant that we were dependent upon others or the local bus system for transportation, severely limiting our freedom to go where and when we wanted. Running errands required planning around bus schedules or waiting until someone could drive us. Anne was sixteen when she got her driver's license, but she hated driving and only took us on short trips to visit Mom's sisters or Dad's brother, all of whom lived in Indiana. I envied my classmates who would return in September with stories about their vacation driving trips out West. How I longed to get out of Muncie and see the world!

From elementary school age until I could drive, I enjoyed considerable freedom on my bike. My parents weren't concerned about me riding alone around the neighborhood or to my piano lessons. Muncie in the 1960s was safe, and I stayed off busy streets. I often rode over to "the field," a three-block, square, empty lot near our house and enjoyed riding on the path that cut through it diagonally. It was bumpy and a challenge to ride, which made it even more fun.

While my bike was useful, I couldn't wait until my legs were long enough to ride the green tandem bicycle that had been parked in our garage since I was about two years old. Dad had wanted a way to enjoy an activity with my brother, John. Dad felt bad that he couldn't do the things that other fathers did, such as playing ball, teaching John to hunt and fish, or taking him camping. I know that John often wished for a dad who could share activities like his friends' fathers; Dad wanted something that they could do together. He found the perfect solution in Indianapolis: a custom-made bicycle built for two. John could steer it in front, and Dad's powerful legs would provide the speed. They rode all over Muncie, with Dad teaching John the street names and basic traffic rules. Dad not only knew each street and which way it went; he knew the location of every stop sign and traffic light. He could even tell if John ran a stop sign!

When my legs finally grew long enough, I took my turn in the front. Dad taught me the same things that he had told my siblings but said that I was the one who was the "speed demon." I loved going fast. It was such a feeling of power that I otherwise never got to experience. Dad didn't complain about having to pump harder. I think that he loved the feeling of motion, too. I'm not sure what happened to that first bike; when I was about ten years old, Dad bought a shiny new red Schwinn tandem with wire baskets and two side mirrors. It was great fun showing it off!

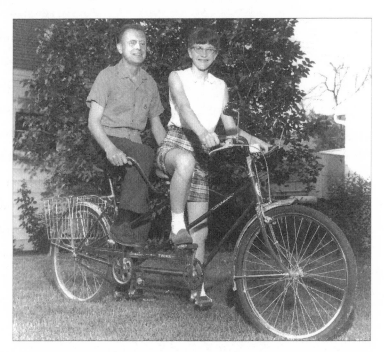

Mario and Mary with the new bike

Looking back, I'm amazed that he was so trusting of us kids. He couldn't see oncoming cars (though he heard them), but he didn't seem to worry about one of us steering into a pothole or being hit by a car. We never had an accident on the tandem, though I do remember many knee scrapes from falling off my own bike.

Ever since I was eight years old, I dreamed of getting my driver's license, that symbol of freedom. The years that I waited seemed endless. All my friends had parents who drove them places; if I wanted to go somewhere, I either walked, rode my bike, or took a bus. If my destination couldn't be reached by one of those modes of transportation, or if I couldn't find a ride, I stayed home. I spent a lot of lonely weekends wishing that I could drive.

Although Anne and John got their driver's licenses at age sixteen, they were only around for a couple of years and then left home for college. While I was glad to go for occasional rides with them, I yearned for my independence. The years crawled by while I waited first for driver's ed and then that glorious day when I got my license! Now I could drive the seven blocks to school on rainy days and even better, take my friends home. I could drive to my evening meetings for Junior Achievement and go to the library whenever I needed instead of shivering on the corner, waiting for the bus. I took Mom to the store whenever she needed to buy groceries or to doctor appointments. She expressed many times to me how grateful she was that she could ride in a car again. She often had painful bladder infections, and I can't imagine how she managed to take the bus to the doctor when she was ill.

Sometimes I drove Dad to evening visitations for deceased acquaintances at funeral homes. Dad knew a lot of people, and he often asked me to take him for a viewing to express his condolences.

I walked with him around the crowded funeral home parlor, waiting patiently while he offered sympathy to the family and sneaking looks at the open coffin.

In the fall of 1970, my senior year in high school, Dad ran for judge of Superior Court. It was the first office that he'd campaigned for since I was born. I'm sure that the sting of losing the mayoral race in 1952 influenced him to leave politics, but as he got older and retirement became more likely, he decided that it would be good to have the steady income that being a judge would provide. He'd also be eligible for a pension, something that he wouldn't have if he stayed with the law firm. Dad not only won the election; he was the top vote-getter. He was sworn into office as Judge of Superior Court on January 1, 1971. After the ceremony, I got to sit in his big leather chair behind the bench and banged the gavel loudly to bring the court to order. Instead of instant quiet and respect, I got scowls from Anne and Mom, which brought my legal career to a quick end.

With almost 70,000 people, Muncie felt confining and boring to my seventeen-year-old self. I knew that there was a larger world to explore, and I was anxious to leave for college. I never considered going to Ball State University. It was nearly in my back yard, and I surely didn't want to spend four more years living at home. I decided that the University of Dayton was the right size, in a city that wasn't too big, and far enough away from Muncie that I felt independent, yet able to drive home in 90 minutes. I didn't think twice about leaving my parents alone. They were perfectly capable of living independently and never made me feel guilty about wanting to leave.

Like Anne, I reveled in walking alone or with friends at college. I wasn't interested in drinking and partying either. My fear of failure prodded me to spend many hours studying and memorizing facts to regurgitate on exams. I worked very hard and earned a 3.9 GPA my first semester. I felt greatly relieved that I could handle my college classes, and although I still was terrified of failing, knew that I would pass.

While I was a sophomore at Dayton, my longtime high school sweetheart, Jeff Harper, asked me to marry him. He was a senior at Brown University in Providence, Rhode Island, and would be going on to graduate school the following summer. We married June 23, 1973, and moved to Charlottesville, Virginia, where he earned his PhD in Pharmacology and I earned my BS in Elementary Education from the University of Virginia.

Five years later, we moved to a townhouse located near Chapel Hill, North Carolina, so Jeff could take a post-doctoral fellowship and conduct research at the University of North Carolina. We loved the ambiance of the old college town; it was beautiful, with lots of activities and events. I envisioned spending the rest of our lives there, figuring that surely, Jeff could find a job at nearby Research Triangle Park, a consortium of large science and technology companies.

Meanwhile, my parents were living alone in our family house on West Jackson Street.

My brother, John, had married and moved to Anderson, about thirty minutes away from Muncie. Anne, divorced with two children, was working on her PhD at Ball State, and Rita was married and living in Wisconsin. I was the farthest away, although we made trips back several times a year and Mom and Dad had visited us in Charlottesville.

In 1978, Dad was approaching 65 and, having served two terms as a County Judge, decided that it was time to retire. Mom was worried about having him "underfoot" all day, thinking that he had few hobbies and would not have enough to do. The winters had become almost unbearable, and a recent blizzard frightened her when Dad became temporarily lost in the snow. She described her fears in a call one day, and I suggested that perhaps they might want to consider moving to North Carolina. We had four seasons, but not as cold and certainly not as much snow. And I'd just learned that I was pregnant with my first child.

I was surprised when my proposal was met with enthusiasm. Could Mom and Dad leave Muncie after spending virtually all their lives there? Both were almost 65; would it be too difficult to get used a new home, learn a new community, or make new friends? Apparently not. They authorized me to find a realtor, and Mom began the process of paring down a lifetime of accumulated possessions in preparation for their move. Dad announced that he would not seek re-election to a shocked community. Plans were made for them to leave Muncie at the end of December 1978 when Dad's term would expire.

The first house that Jeff and I toured was perfect for them. It was a one story, with two bedrooms, two baths, and a large living room. Best of all was the screened-in porch located off both the living room and master bedroom. They could sit out on the porch, feel the gentle breeze, and listen to the birds singing. The house was on a large, wooded lot located on a quiet street across from a golf course. Even better, Dad could walk with Mattie, his seeing eye dog, to a neighborhood drug store, small grocery store, and bank. Mom and Dad wouldn't be totally relying on me to run errands for them.

It took them about ten minutes to decide to make an offer on the house, literally buying it sight unseen. Mom and Dad always trusted me, whether with their lives when I was 16 and driving or spending tens of thousands of their money on a house. Although I'd never given them a reason not to trust me, it still took a huge amount of courage to buy their first house since 1950 and move across the country where Jeff and I were the only people that they knew.

They arrived in Chapel Hill January 2, 1979. Jeff and I (with a large pregnant belly) helped them unpack and familiarized them with the layout of the house. Our daughter was born about three weeks later, on the 19th, much to everyone's delight. Both of my parents loved Katie. They were thrilled to hold her, bouncing her gently and making silly faces and noises. When Katie was about a month old, we didn't hesitate to have Mom and Dad babysit for us. It never occurred to me to worry about their ability to care for her. After all, they'd successfully raised four children.

Life was good. My parents adjusted easily to their new home and began making new friends at church and in the neighborhood. They took adult leisure classes and went to plays and concerts with friends. I'd go to their house and pay bills while they entertained Katie. Other times, I'd put Katie in her car seat and take Mom and Dad for rides or go on errands. I loved living in the small college town; it was especially nice having my parents so close. It was a joy to watch them play with their granddaughter. Little did I know that our time together would be limited.

• • • •
• •

BIG CHANGES

LATE ON A March afternoon, Jeff arrived home from the lab, took off his coat, and came into the kitchen where I was giving Katie her dinner. He kissed me hello, then smiled at his daughter and said, "Hi, Katie! What's for dinner?"

"Cookie!" She grinned up at her daddy.

"You're not eating a cookie! That's a banana!"

Katie squished the piece of banana with her fingers and smiled looking up for his reaction.

"Oh you're my silly one. Would you like some more milk?"

While getting the milk carton from the refrigerator, Jeff casually turned to me and said, "Well, I have some news. Alton [his mentor and boss] has been offered a job in Houston. He'll be the department chair at the University of Texas Health Science Center."

"Oh, that's interesting," I said.

"And he wants me to come with him. I would be an Assistant Professor of Internal Medicine and Pharmacology. It would mean a good salary and my own lab. I'd get to teach Pharmacology to med students, too."

Stunned at the news, I was less than enthusiastic. "What? You mean leave Chapel Hill? We just moved into this house nine months ago. What about my parents? How could I leave them and take their beloved grandchild?" I tried not to sound upset. I didn't want Katie to catch my fear and disappointment. "Can't you get a job here in the Research Triangle? There's lots of technical jobs there and we wouldn't have to move."

"I don't want to work in industry. I want to be in a university or medical school where I can do my own research. Alton is going to Houston in a couple of weeks. He wants us to come with him. I'll have some interviews and you can look at houses."

I was devastated. Worst of all, it appeared that I had no choice in the matter. I would follow my husband to a sprawling city where I knew no one and would have no support raising our daughter. I'd never lived in a big city and had no idea what to expect. All I knew about Houston was that it full of violent crime, unbearably hot and humid, and had monstrous, traffic-clogged freeways. Moving to the big city from the idyllic Chapel Hill terrified me.

Mom and Dad took the news better than I expected. They offered to babysit Katie for the weekend, and I didn't think twice about leaving my seventeen-month-old with Mom and Dad for the spring weekend that we flew to Houston to find a house. After all, they'd raised four children and were thrilled to have their granddaughter stay with them.

Upon our return, Katie ran to greet us with a big smile and twinkling eyes, with Mom following close behind.

While hugging Katie, I asked Mom how things had gone.

"Oh, she was just perfect! We had so much fun with her. We played and she took naps, and we just had a fine time."

Dad came into the room and added, "Oh yes! Katie was such a good girl. You know, she does love my dog, Mattie. We'd put her in her highchair and give her some Cheerios. Pretty soon,

I'd hear Mattie go over to the highchair. I wondered what she was doing there and then I heard, 'uh oh!' and some crunching. I realized that Katie was dropping Cheerios down for the dog! She thought that it was so funny to watch the dog eat those Cheerios. She'd laugh and laugh."

"Well, Dad, you wouldn't let us ever feed a dog from the table."

"I know, but she's such a cute little thing, and it didn't really hurt anything."

Dad's response surprised me, since Dad had always enforced strict rules about his dogs.

Although my daughter's dropping Cheerios from her highchair was similar behavior to my brother's when he was that age, Dad didn't seem worried that Mattie would become too attached to Katie, as Baron had to my brother. I noticed that as Dad got older, he relaxed more around the dogs, although they were never allowed on the furniture. His last two dogs—Job, a golden retriever and Admiral, a yellow Labrador—were much loved and almost became pets. Mom took an interest in both dogs and developed a daily routine. Admiral reminded her every morning at 11:00 that it was time for his Milk-Bone treat and circled her, excitedly wagging his tail as Mom made her way to the kitchen.

Mom and Dad talked for days about how much they'd enjoyed having Katie at their house, describing in detail what they had done together. Although I was delighted that her visit had worked out so well, it only made me sadder, realizing that I'd be taking Katie away in only a few weeks.

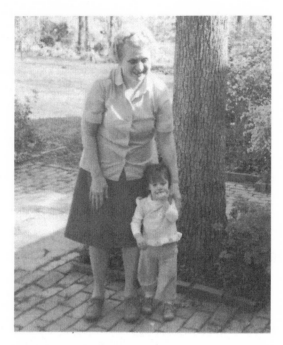

Jane and Katie, 1980

Although Mom and Dad reassured me several times that they had lived on their own for many years before I was born and would manage okay without me, I still felt terribly guilty for leaving them only a year after their move to North Carolina. I'd miss seeing them and wondered who would take them to doctor appointments, the store, or pay their bills. And I was saddened that Katie would not grow up with grandparents nearby.

Their friends and neighbors took up the slack, offering rides to appointments, church, and the grocery store. One person put a help wanted notice up on a bulletin board at the University advertising for someone to read mail and pay bills once a week. The young sorority girl who answered the ad turned into a trusted friend who, when she graduated, found another girl from her sorority who would take her place. My parents kept in contact with all their "girls" for years afterward, delighting in their Christmas cards.

To help relieve my guilt about leaving my parents behind in Chapel Hill, Katie and I flew back to visit them several times during that first year. Jeff was working and couldn't go with us; I have no idea how I managed a squirmy toddler, stroller, luggage, and car seat by myself. Mom and Dad were always happy to see us and excited to play with their granddaughter; I was glad to help out with errands and things around the house.

When my second child, Andrew, was born in October 1981, Mom and Dad flew down to Houston and helped me care for both children. Mom, especially, loved babies and enjoyed holding Andrew and making funny faces to entertain him. As Katie and Andrew grew, my parents taught them how to interact with them. If Katie held up a doll for her grandmother to admire, she instructed Katie to put the doll into her hands so she could feel the doll's face and clothes. "Oh! She has on such a pretty dress. What color is it, Katie?" Both grandchildren quickly learned the rule that I'd grown up with: never leave your toys on the floor where Grandma or Grandpa could step on them!

I always felt a little sad that it was harder for my children to enjoy my parents. Mom couldn't drive my children to the park, or take them out for ice cream, or play Candyland. In contrast, Jeff's parents lived in Maine and Florida, with swimming pools and the beach to entertain them. Jeff's mother took the kids to museums and enjoyed taking Katie shopping. Every night that we visited, she read a book to Katie and Andrew before bedtime. My parents could do none of those things. But they were good listeners and always showed an interest in their grandchildren's activities, whether it be admiring preschool artwork (What colors did you use, Katie?) or listening to Andrew play the guitar as a teenager.

July 21,

Happy Birthday! Rita,

Hope this will be one of the nicest birthdays you ever had. We think of all of you often and wish there weren't so many miles between us.

It was good talking with you a while back and will be calling you again soon. Hope Erica is rid of her problem and that you like your work.

Things are going smoothly for us even though Mary is gone. Our neighbors and friends are really helpful and quite friendly. I grosery shop with the man that drives us to Church. And a friend of your dad's invites him out shopping occasionally. Others have offer us trips to the shopping center so actually we are doing well enough. On the Fourth we ate out with another couple abd had a real nice visit with them. Also that week went to the Village Theater to see live South Pacific. There was a lot of good music and very good acting.

I told you I ripped out my shawl and did it all over. I like the looks of it much better now. About two more rows and it will be finished. It is not quite perfect, but the next one will be considerably better. It just seems to take practice.

Your Aunt Irma has had her operation and I believe is back home.1 She now has an artificial knee besides her two artificial hip bones.

```
        Your dad is feeling good.  He still
swims three times a week and does a lot
of walking.  Aug. sixteenth he goes to
Morristown for a new dog.  Mattie is really
sweet and sometimes downright affectionage
and loveable, but she has a lot of ailments.
She doesn't like to go much either--when
we start out she often tries to turn around
and come back home.
        I met a new friend last week, and she
and I take walks several evenings a week.  It
has been very hot here, but we have been
getting rain which helps a little.  Every-
thing grows like in the tropics.  There is
always something blooming which smells so
sweet.  We get a lot of compliments on our
yard.
        You mentioned towels you needed so
if you like buy some with this birthday
money.  It won't buy much but itss fun to
have some mad money.
        We think of you often and will be
glad to hear how you all are getting along.
        Bye,

        With love,

                Mother
```

Rita showed me that letter many years later. Mom and Dad were always cheerful on the phone after we left Chapel Hill, but I was never sure if they were just trying to reassure me or if they were covering up their difficulties. Apparently, they were doing quite well, and I hadn't needed to suffer guilty thoughts for many years.

•• •
 ••

GIVING UP

WHEN MOM BEGAN failing in her early eighties, it became clear that the house and cooking were becoming too much for her. Dad had few housekeeping skills and was unable to take over her chores. He could open a can of soup or make a peanut butter sandwich, but he couldn't cook on a regular basis. He worried how he'd care for her if she had a stroke or otherwise became incapacitated.

Arthritis in both her knees had eroded the joints so that bones rubbed on bones, causing her constant pain and limiting her movements. Walking, sweeping the floor, and standing to cook dinner all became difficult. Mom also suffered from Paget's disease, which caused bones in her lower spine to grow too quickly and become deformed, pressing on nerves and causing pain.

When she was diagnosed in her late fifties, medication helped, as did back surgery a few years later. Yet the strong pain medication that she took for decades and her barely controlled high blood pressure combined to decrease her kidney functions.

Mom's hearing progressively declined, but she would not admit it. I can still hear her say, "Mario! Speak up! You're mumbling again." She was adamant that he had a hearing problem and was glad when Dad got his hearing aids, but she refused to acknowledge that she needed her own pair. In a reversal of roles—Mom had begged Dad to get artificial eyes—Dad frequently told her that she'd benefit from hearing aids. Mom didn't appreciate the irony. Dad told me several times about how terrified he was of losing his hearing. How would he communicate without his sight or hearing? And losing the ability to hear his beloved classical music was unthinkable.

Helplessly watching her slow physical and mental decline, he didn't know what to do. Their lives had gone well as long as both were healthy; they functioned perfectly as a couple. But one without the other was inconceivable.

Hiring a full-time caregiver would be too expensive and would drain their resources quickly. Dad still worried about money, but more importantly, neither wanted an outsider to watch them 24/7 and would possibly cause more problems than they would solve. Privacy and independence were extremely important to them, and the idea of having someone in the house, perhaps judging them or talking too much, was not acceptable. They preferred to read, listen to music, and chat among themselves—not have to keep up a conversation with a stranger.

After many phone conversations between my siblings and parents, it became obvious that a change had to be made. They could no longer live on their own. The only option seemed to be an assisted living facility, where they'd have help if needed, yet be mostly independent. Deciding upon a location was the next problem. My siblings all lived in the cold Midwest. Mom and Dad enjoyed the temperate climate in North Carolina and didn't want to go back to the snow and ice.

I offered to help them find an assisted living facility in Houston. Meals would be provided, staff would be close by, and I could take them out for errands, doctor appointments, or to my house for a home-cooked meal. They gratefully accepted my offer, and in August 1998 moved to Houston to a facility just minutes from my home.

It wasn't easy for them to give up their perfect home in the beautiful town of Chapel Hill to transition to institutional living at Brighton Gardens in Houston. They moved into a small studio apartment that was cooled by a noisy air conditioner. They needed fresh air, but it was usually much too hot to open the window, and even on nice days, traffic noise from the street and nearby freeway was an annoying presence. I knew that they missed their porch; just being confined to one room together with their last dog, Admiral, had to have been almost suffocating.

I did everything that I could to make the transition easier. Once a week, I collected their laundry to wash at home. Mom didn't trust the staff to do it properly and Dad didn't want to pay extra for the service. I didn't mind the additional laundry; I figured that Mom had spent years washing my clothes, so it was the least that I could do for her.

Every week, I took them out for rides to explore Houston. Dad wanted to know the names of major streets, and at red lights he frequently asked, "Where are we? Which direction does Westheimer go?" We often combined our drives with running errands; they were happy to just get out of that confining room. Sometimes we had lunch at my house—they enjoyed my simple sandwiches—which were a treat for them after eating institutional food every day. After taking them home, I read their mail to them and paid the bills.

Occasionally, Jeff and I took them for outings to area state parks or Galveston. They enjoyed the quiet of Brazos Bend State Park and even held a baby alligator at the park's Nature Center. I can still hear Dad inhaling the salty fresh air while standing next to the Gulf of Mexico. Mom had severe arthritis in both of her knees and couldn't walk far. But she enjoyed riding in her wheelchair on trails or going into the shops on the Galveston Strand.

When Anne came down for a visit, we went on the City of Houston boat tour down the Houston Ship Channel. We described the huge cargo ships docked along the route and attempted to describe what the oil refineries looked like. They loved the ride and the screeching of the seagulls following the boat.

Every Sunday, I brought them over for a home-cooked meal made by my husband, Jeff. Afterward, Jeff read the local *Houston Chronicle* newspaper to Dad while Mom often fell asleep in my comfortable overstuffed leather chair.

In the summer, they liked to sit out by the pool, enjoying the slightly cooler evening air, while Admiral watched our dog, Goldy, jump into the water. Admiral was unusual for a retriever—he wouldn't follow Goldy's joyful leap to retrieve a floating toy. Once, Admiral slipped into the pool and just slapped at the water with his paws. It was obvious that he didn't know how to swim, so I jumped in and guided him to the steps. He seemed so humiliated—poor dog—and gave the pool a wide berth after that incident. Dad was surprised that he was afraid of the water and surmised that perhaps he'd had some training at the Seeing Eye to discourage water play.

I didn't mind devoting so much time to my parents. I'd happily quit my stressful job, knowing that caring for them would be an almost full-time job in itself. I finally felt at peace with myself. I felt that by helping them now, I was making up for leaving them behind in Chapel Hill twenty years earlier.

•• •

SAYING GOODBYE

FROM THE TIME they moved to Houston in 1998, both parents had frequent doctor appointments, but Mom's health began to deteriorate rapidly. Years of high blood pressure and painkillers for the unrelenting pain of Paget's disease and osteoarthritis took their toll. Her knees were both severely inflamed and swollen, making walking extremely painful and necessitating using a wheelchair when she needed to walk further than a few feet.

She developed symptoms of kidney failure: fatigue, swollen legs, and confusion. We went to a nephrologist, a kidney specialist, who did numerous tests and prescribed medications but was unable to prevent further damage.

Her last appointment with the nephrologist was in early June. He told her frankly that the only option available was dialysis. She quickly and firmly replied, "No, I don't want to do that."

I wasn't surprised by her decision. Mom knew of other Brighton Gardens residents who went to dialysis several times a week, and she'd said before that she didn't want to put herself through such torment.

We arrived back at their room, where Dad sat listening to the radio. Upon hearing us enter, he turned off the news and stood to greet us. He was anxious to hear what the doctor had said but waited until

Mom was seated in her usual gold fabric lounge chair. After stowing her wheelchair, I sat on the floor next to Admiral, who was lying at Dad's feet. I stroked Admiral's handsome wide head and fondled his floppy ears while I listened to my parents' conversation.

"What did the doctor say?" asked Dad.

"That I need dialysis," Mom said bluntly. "But I told him that I didn't want to do that."

Dad inhaled sharply, his face stricken, as if he couldn't believe that Mom didn't want to fight the disease.

"Mom," I said, "you know what that means if you don't have dialysis."

"It means that I'll die," she said in a matter-of-fact tone.

"Yes, it does. It doesn't sound like a very pleasant death, either. Without your kidneys working, you'll slowly be poisoned by your own waste," I explained.

"Well, I don't want to be tied to a machine. I'm ready to go. I've had a good life. I'm eighty-five years old. Nobody in my family has ever lived past eighty, so it's my turn."

Looking up at my mother, I was surprised at how calm she appeared. Her fair skin, with almost no wrinkles, was smooth. No grimacing or frowning. No tears, no choked voice.

I glanced at Dad's face. The reality of losing his beloved Jane was sinking in; I'd never seen him look so sad. His face was contorted as he tried not to cry. He exhaled a heavy sigh.

There was no more discussion. She had made her decision. Dad didn't try to convince her to go on dialysis; he knew that she was firm.

"Mom, we'll do whatever it takes to make you as comfortable as possible. The doctor gave me hospice information. I'll call them this afternoon."

Houston Hospice came the next day and ordered all the necessary equipment and supplies. Anne, John, and Rita flew down to Houston to help me care for her. Yet, even with round-the-clock shifts shared among the four of us, we realized that we couldn't provide all the care that she needed. We were unable to relieve her pain and misery. The hospice nurse recommended their inpatient unit; we were relieved that she would get excellent twenty-four hour care and hoped that they would be able to control her pain.

Dad stayed with her for hours every day, often lying beside her and holding her hand. He listened attentively to her breathing, noting minute changes. On the evening of July 2, he said to me, "Mary, I'm going to stay here tonight with Jane. I'll call you if I need you."

"Ok, Dad." I felt bad about leaving them but knew that he needed some privacy. "I'll take Admiral out tonight. Jeff says that he's doing just fine at our house."

"Thank you." He turned his head back to my mother and breathed out a long, forlorn sigh.

The phone rang at 2:00 a.m., awakening me from a fitful sleep. I grabbed it and heard Dad say, "Mary, she's gone."

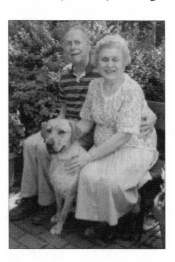

Mario, Jane, and Admiral
Chapel Hill, NC 1992

$$\bullet\bullet \quad \bullet$$
$$\bullet \quad \bullet\bullet$$

LIFE ALONE

AFTER WE RETURNED from Mom's funeral in Muncie, Dad's first request was to move to an even smaller room. There were too many painful memories lurking. He wanted to start fresh and asked me to remove her clothing and possessions. I fought back tears as I packed away her things and wondered if Dad was callous—how could he want to live in a place with no reminders of his wife of fifty-eight years? Now, I realize that his memories were all locked in his brain; photos were meaningless, and the faint lingering smell of her perfume was painful to breathe.

Dad adjusted to life alone at Brighton Gardens. Lonely female residents found him to be a good listener; he enjoyed their conversations to a point but was always happy to escape back to the comfort of his room. When he wasn't listening to the Houston Public Radio station, he read Talking Books on tape from the Texas State Library. When he turned ninety, he announced that he was going to re-read Greek mythology just for fun.

He also enjoyed membership in the Cassette Tape Club. Members recorded letters and sent them to one person, who in turn listened, commented, and forwarded it on to the next in line. Not all the members were blind, but all liked to talk into a tape recorder and tell jokes, play music, or discuss current events.

Admiral provided comfort and a schedule that gave structure to his day. Every morning Dad fed him, then took him outside for his morning walk. Just before lunch, Admiral got a snack and again went out for a short walk. Dad usually went for a brisk afternoon walk with him, following the sidewalks inside the property. He had quickly memorized the layout soon after arriving at the facility and had no difficulty finding his way around the grounds. He chose not to walk outside of the gates, saying that Houston traffic was too loud and dangerously fast. Unlike Chapel Hill, it was not a walkable neighborhood with nearby businesses or quiet neighborhoods to explore.

I tried to spend as much time as I could with Dad, continuing to take him and Admiral on errands two or three times a week. I was surprised at how much easier it was without Mom and felt rather guilty for thinking it. I hadn't realized how much extra time and energy the routine took: waiting for her to get ready, pushing the wheelchair down to the main entrance, helping her get into the car, and finally stowing the wheelchair. Now I simply called Dad to let him know that I was leaving my house, and he said without fail, "Okay, I'll meet you downstairs." By the time I arrived, he was patiently standing next to the driveway. One blazing summer day, I was a few minutes late. As usual, Dad stood in the sun with Admiral lying on the hot cement next to him.

"Dad, you should wait in the shade. It's too hot to be standing out here."

"Oh, it doesn't bother me at all. I like it," he said as he settled into the front seat. "Come, Admiral!"

The big yellow lab didn't need a second command. He jumped in and curled up under the dashboard. Dad patted him and found his tail, making sure that it was tucked safely under the dog's body before closing the car door.

"See how warm he is? His old bones just love that Texas sun."

I reached over and felt his soft coat. "Wow, he's hot. I just don't want either of you to get overheated. Sorry that I'm a little late."

"Oh, we don't mind at all. I was listening to those old blue jays. They were really squawking at something. They must have a nest close by."

"Yes, there's a magnolia tree right across the driveway. That's probably where they were—maybe they didn't like Admiral. Do you want to go to the bank first?" I asked as I drove out the gate.

Although I now had more free time, I had no intention of returning to a paying job. I was president of a nonprofit, the Fibromyalgia Association of Houston, and that kept me as busy as I wanted to be. We were all volunteers, and I joked at every meeting that, "If you don't like the job I'm doing, feel free to cut my salary in half." I also suffered from fibromyalgia, although medication and exercise helped to keep my symptoms of pain and fatigue under control. I was blessed that Jeff's income was sufficient, as a full-time job would have been impossible for me. Running the organization from my home gave me a purpose in life, yet if I got tired and needed a nap, nobody complained. I liked the flexibility and knowing that I was helping others cope with their illness.

I enjoyed spending time with Dad. I got to know him in a completely different way, not just as a daughter, but seeing him in a new light, without my mother's influence. I wanted to know him as a person, not just roll my eyes when he repeated his stories of long-ago times. And I was grateful to have this opportunity. He was eighty-five when Mom died; I decided to make the most of whatever time he had left. He still had an adventuresome spirit and a stunning intellect. I was not going to let him rot in a small room at Brighton Gardens.

While most of their first year in Houston was devoted to Mom and her failing health, Dad also had worrisome symptoms. He had survived surgery for stage two colon cancer six years earlier; now at his advanced age, he would not need further treatment. However, his blood chemistry was consistently abnormal, and his doctor referred him to M. D. Anderson Cancer Center for further tests. He was diagnosed with splenic lymphoma and given a new chemotherapy that had surprisingly few side effects.

We went to Anderson for monthly bloodwork and doctor appointments. Cancer hospital waiting rooms are filled with anxious, very ill patients, but when Admiral curled up at Dad's feet, people smiled, and the tension began to ease. Inevitably, someone would come over to say hello and ask permission to pet the dog. Dad gently refused and explained why. So many people wanted to pet him, including doctors in hospital elevators who reached out and petted Admiral without asking, that I made a bright red sign for his harness: *Working Dog. Please do not touch!* Seeing eye dogs become distracted if pet by strangers and may not notice a car or a step. Although that wasn't a problem when Dad walked with me, we still wanted to educate the public about the necessity of resisting the temptation to pet a guide dog.

Dad didn't let his cancer interrupt his exercise routine. He used small hand weights in his room and took part in chair exercises with other residents in the morning class. In the summers, he liked to swim in our backyard pool. I taught him some water aerobics; after our sessions, he often said how "invigorated" he felt. Dad was proud of his strength and endurance, and a firm believer in exercising both the body and mind.

I could keep him busy, but I couldn't fill the void left by Mom. He needed someone his own age, a peer, to share confidences and worries. Since he left Muncie, Dad had kept in contact with his former secretary and court reporter, Frances Middleton. When both were widowed, the telephone calls became more frequent. Dad began asking me to book flights to Indiana, ostensibly to visit Anne at her rural home, but I suspected that he was most interested in spending a day with Frances. The friendship grew into love. They discussed marriage, but Frances didn't want to leave her family and move to Houston, and Dad couldn't move back to Muncie. Daily phone calls and trips to Indiana sustained their relationship; I offered to take care of Frances if she wanted to move here, but she was fearful of becoming a burden on me.

Three years after his lymphoma diagnosis, Dad developed severe Type 2 diabetes. It was a shock to both of us, as Dad was not overweight and ate a healthy diet. After a week's hospitalization, he was released and referred to the Lighthouse of Houston, an organization that works with blind people and offers diabetes education and management services. He needed to learn how to test his blood sugar and give himself insulin shots.

Dad was determined to do everything that the doctor recommended, following every direction to the letter. He had me read labels and counted sugars. He switched to no sugar added ice cream and artificially sweetened candy and closely monitored his diet.

We went to the Lighthouse several times, where we learned about the importance of diet and what to do if the blood sugar level was too low. The instructor patiently taught him how to use a lancet to prick his finger and how to get his blood onto the test strip. She explained how the glucose meter worked and how to insert the test strip. The machine announced the reading, and he wrote the value down in Braille. Once he mastered testing, he learned how to insert the insulin injection into his abdomen. I was surprised at how quickly he memorized the many steps involved with testing and injecting—I would have been constantly referring to the printed material.

Understanding what he needed to do didn't mean that he could easily carry it out physically. Dad had an essential tremor, which meant that his hand shook, especially when bringing food to his mouth. Food fell off his fork or soup splashed out of his spoon. His coffee cup shook, and I worried that he'd be burned. The tremor wasn't serious, but it was certainly annoying, and at times, embarrassing.

Each time he needed to check his blood levels (four times a day at first), it seemed to take him a long time to get all the supplies together. He painstakingly gathered the meter, lancet, test strips, alcohol wipes, used needle container, and insulin injections. He methodically arranged each item so he knew where to find it and then slowly got up to wash his hands.

Finally returning to the table, he sat down and prepared to lance his finger. After working to open the small alcohol pad and cleansing the spot on his finger, he carefully loaded the lance with the sharp needle. His hand wavered as he guided the instrument toward his left index finger. Satisfied that was in the correct position, he pushed the button and felt for the blood to ooze out. Many times, he failed to get blood and was forced to stick himself again. I felt terrible as he made yet another attempt to prick his finger. But Dad was determined. He had been persistent his whole life, always working harder than a sighted person; otherwise, he would have spent his life sitting in a chair, being waited on. He had been always independent, and he was not going to allow someone else to test his blood or give him his medicine, even when it would have been easier and sometimes less painful.

I tried to rein in my impatience as he moved slowly. It seemed that he often had to check his blood just before going somewhere; I offered to help, to which he usually said, "I can do it." If he had a particularly difficult time pricking his finger, and we were in a hurry, he sometimes gave in and allowed me to lance him.

Injecting insulin seemed to be easier. He just needed to clean the injection site and hold the syringe at the proper angle to his abdomen. The action didn't require as fine of motor coordination as lancing the finger.

"Doesn't that hurt, Dad?" I asked as he plunged the syringe into his flesh. "No, not really. It doesn't bother me at all."

I shuddered as I watched him pull the needle out. I was surprised that he could be so casual about injecting himself. I tried to imagine myself doing that several times a day and prayed that I'd never get diabetes.

Being diabetic and eighty-eight years old didn't stop Dad from traveling. He carefully packed all his supplies in his carry-on bag and faithfully monitored his health. He continued to fly with Admiral several times a year to Indiana to visit Anne and Frances. Anne told me how sad and frustrated she felt as she watched him try to prick his finger. As he grew older, the tremor worsened, yet he rarely asked for help.

When Jeff and I took him on trips, we needed to allow plenty of time for dad to take care of his needs. Whether it was checking his blood sugar levels or going for a walk, everything took more time than I imagined. Dad walked slower and slower. It was a hard adjustment for me since he had always been a fast walker. As a child, I hurried to keep up with him, feeling grown up and excited to be walking with my dad. I was saddened though, as he grew older and frailer, knowing that he would continue deteriorating. I gained still more patience when I slowed down to match his pace.

Despite the extra physical and emotional energy required to successfully navigate through each portion of a trip, I continued to plan vacations because I knew how much Dad enjoyed the fresh air, visiting with friends and relatives, and getting away from his small, institutional room. Jeff and I loved traveling; while taking Dad with us required extra planning and patience, it wasn't a sacrifice to include him. We took him with us to Orange County, California, where we visited our daughter Katie and went for short walks on the beach. He enjoyed breathing in the fresh Pacific Ocean air from a bench perched high on a cliff while listening to the sound of waves breaking on the rocks below. We explored the River Walk in San Antonio, picked up shells on Sanibel Island, Florida, and spent a week in the rainforest of Belize. He marveled at the tropical birds singing outside our cabin, enjoyed a day exploring Mayan ruins, and relished the silence of a cave while riding in a canoe. He clicked his tongue often to gauge the height of the cave; he was uncannily correct in pronouncing dimensions of the tunnels and caverns.

The summer that Dad was ninety-one, we stayed at a condo for a week in Park City, Utah. He delighted in breathing in the fresh mountain air; he enjoyed the crisp breezes which provided relief from the heat and humidity of Houston. One day we went for a drive in the mountains and stopped at a trail near the road. While Dad enjoyed riding in cars, getting out and exploring nature was much more interesting. Uneven paths didn't stop him. He took my arm and I simply paused when we came to a rock or root and said, "Watch out, there's a big root here that you'll need to step over." He lifted his foot up high and off we went.

Trees fascinated Dad. He liked to touch their bark and feel the shape of their leaves. He knew the names of many by touch, just as he knew the names of birds by their song. If we happened upon a particularly large, old tree, I'd stop and have him try to put his arms around it—like he used to do when we were kids. I think that Dad was the original "tree hugger."

"Whoa! I can't even put my arms all the way around it. This must be an ancient tree. How far apart are my hands? This thing must be nine feet in circumference!"

As we continued on the trail, I stopped by a pile of melting snow that was still on the mountain, despite the warmth of that June day. Since I've lived in Houston for over 40 years, snow is a rarity for me and I'm always excited to find some.

"Hey Dad! Here's some snow! I can't believe that there's still some here. It's just down at your feet."

He reached down and grabbed a handful. He made a snowball, grinned, and started to throw it at me.

"Hey, stop! I've got to get a picture," I said as I quickly pulled the camera out of my bag. "Okay, now you can throw it."

The snowball landed just feet away from me, but I got the shot. Dad's red polo shirt and khaki pants stood in contrast to the background of snow and pine trees. He's holding the snowball with both hands, a sly grin on his face as he anticipates throwing a snowball for the first time in many years. It turned out to be one of my favorite photos ever taken of him.

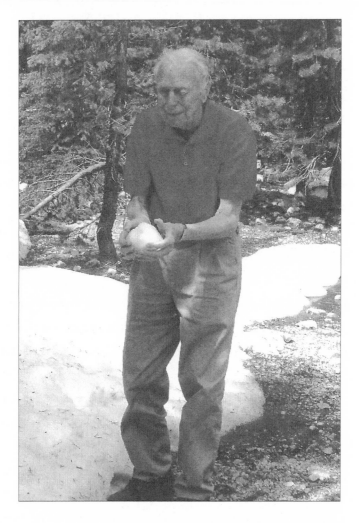

•••

ADMIRAL

ON MOST OF his trips with us, Dad didn't need to bring
Admiral. He could walk with us, and taking care of the dog would
have been too much. The big yellow lab boarded at the vet's kennel.
I know that he would have loved going along, but Dad was firm.
I suspect that he relished some time without the responsibilities of
tending a dog.

In August 2002, after a week in Colorado where Dad enjoyed
many hours listening to a rushing mountain stream next to our
cottage, we picked up Admiral at the kennel. All seemed normal as
I dropped them off at the entrance to Brighton Gardens and drove
home. While unpacking later that evening, the phone rang. Glancing
at the Caller ID, I was surprised that it was Dad. He didn't usually
call after dinner.

"Mary, something is wrong with Admiral. I think he's dying."

"What? But we just picked him up at the vet's. He looked fine."

"Well, after you dropped us off, we came up to the room as usual.
I removed his harness and he lay down in his corner. I didn't pay any
attention to him because he always naps when there isn't much going
on. But I just tried to take him out to do his business and when
I called him, he didn't respond. I thought he was just tired from being

boarded and he was sleeping it off. Then I just went to him and petted him, but he still didn't respond. Something is very wrong."

"I'll be right over."

Still in disbelief that Admiral was very ill, I drove as fast as I dared down Bellaire Boulevard. That portion of the road is well-known for being a speed trap, and I rehearsed in my mind what I'd say to the Southside Place police officer if I was pulled over. The Stoplight Gods were with me, no police cars were hiding, and I made it to Brighton Gardens in record time.

Not waiting for the elevator, I took the stairs two steps at a time and walked quickly down the hall to Dad's room. I knocked once, opened the door, and saw Admiral lying stretched out on the floor next to his master's bed.

"Hi, Dad," I said as I crossed the room and knelt by the beautiful yellow lab. "Hey Admiral, how ya doin'?" I said quietly as I patted his head and gently rubbed his floppy ears.

Dad repeated what he'd told me over the phone while I noticed the dog's lethargy and lack of response.

"You're right, Dad. Something is definitely wrong. I think that I should call the vet."

"Well, it's 7:30. She won't still be at the office."

"I know, but one time she gave me her cell phone number. Let me try calling."

I was relieved when Dr. Frei answered the phone. After a short conversation, she asked if we would like her to come down to see Admiral. Fortunately, she lived only 10 minutes away, and soon she was examining him.

"How old is he?" asked the vet. "He looks like he has some years on him."

"He's twelve," answered Dad.

"Without all my equipment, I can't really tell what's wrong, but he needs to go to the emergency clinic tonight. They can run some tests and make a diagnosis," she explained.

Admiral was too ill to walk and too heavy for us to carry. I remembered the luggage cart down in the lobby, ran downstairs, and soon we had Admiral loaded into my SUV.

When we arrived at the emergency hospital 15 minutes later, I hurried inside to get some help. I was grateful to learn that Dr. Frei had called ahead and told them to expect us. Almost immediately, two techs brought a stainless steel cart out to the car and carefully unloaded the motionless dog. We watched as they disappeared behind the examining room door, and we settled into the uncomfortable, hard, plastic chairs to wait.

Neither of us felt like talking. I didn't want to read aloud as I normally would to pass the time. We sat together but alone in our thoughts and fears. Dad heavily sighed several times; his face was drawn with worry. I wondered how he would manage without his beloved dog. More than guiding him around dangerous objects, Admiral was a companion, particularly since Mom's death three years before. Dad took comfort in his presence, feeling the dog's weight against his feet and legs or talking to him during the course of the day. "Admiral, let's get your harness on. It's time for your walk." Admiral provided a structure and routine to the day, allowing Dad to focus on another living being and offering a distraction from grieving for Mom.

But now Dad faced another potential major loss, and my heart ached for him. I felt my own sorrow. I couldn't imagine life without Admiral. He and my dog, Goldy, got along very well and enjoyed playing together. Anne and I had often wondered who would die first: Dad or Admiral. If Admiral survived my Dad, we'd have a family fight on our hands. Anne, John, and I all wanted him. Now it seemed that argument would never happen. While I was relieved that he would outlive Admiral, I felt a deep sadness for Dad grieving again, totally alone in the room without the comfort of his dog.

Finally, at about midnight, the vet came to the door and invited us back to the examining room.

"Well, we've done a CT scan and bloodwork on Admiral. I'm afraid that he has two very aggressive and malignant tumors on his spleen. One has burst and released a lot of blood, so he's very anemic now."

"Can you do surgery?" I asked.

"We could, but I don't think that it would prolong his life more than a few weeks. He's twelve years old, and that's the normal life span for a big dog. I think that the surgery would be very hard on him, and he wouldn't be his old self."

A small gasp escaped from Dad's lips as his brain processed the news. I felt a lump grow in my throat and thoughts swirled. How could this be happening? He'd been just fine! Thank God this didn't happen while we were in Colorado, but it should never happen. Admiral should just live forever and die when Dad passes. The thought of separating them was too painful for me to contemplate.

"Do you want to take him home?"

"No. It was too hard to get him here. We'd never get him home by ourselves," answered Dad. "No," he sighed, "just keep him. If he gets a lot worse, you can do something."

"All right. Would you like to come back in the morning and pick him up?" the vet asked, looking at me. "You can take him directly to your regular vet."

He didn't have to say, "to be put to sleep." We knew that there were no options. Admiral was clearly suffering. In the morning, his pain would cease.

Dad and I drove home in silence. Without his dog, I had to walk with him back to his room. No longer could I just drop Dad and Admiral off at the main entrance and continue on my way.

The following morning, I went back to the emergency clinic. A different set of techs gingerly and respectfully loaded Admiral into the back of my SUV and gently closed the tailgate. With tears in my eyes, I drove down the freeway to pick up Dad. It would be Admiral's last ride. How he loved to go for rides! But this morning he lay quietly where they placed him in the back. I hoped that he was still enjoying the ride.

When we arrived at Dr. Frei's clinic, again two techs came with a rolling cart and took him inside. We exchanged brief greetings with the staff and were escorted to a small back room where we could spend as much time as we needed with Admiral.

Dad sat on a chair with Admiral on the floor next to him. Dad stroked his head, speaking softly to him, telling him what a good boy he was and how much he'd miss him. Admiral struggled to sit up and managed to put his head on Dad's knee, causing Dad to gasp when he felt the weight of Admiral's head. His voice choked up as he fought back tears. My tears streamed uncontrollably down my cheeks; I cried silently, not wanting to interfere with their final goodbye. Admiral slid back down to the floor, unable to sustain a sitting position.

"Dad, are you ready? Dr. Frei is here."

"Yes, go ahead. I don't want him to suffer anymore."

She gave him the shot. Dad reached down and held him with both hands. He didn't feel any quiver or movement; Admiral just "slipped away."

Minutes later, we left with only his leash.

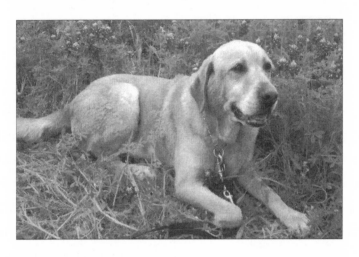

∴∵

WALKING ALONE

DAD WAS QUIET during the short ride back to Brighton Gardens, though he did mention that he now needed a cane. He was worried about walking around the assisted living complex. It was no problem for him to walk alone to the dining room and main living area, but he was afraid of running into an elderly person and perhaps knocking them over. A cane would make it easier for the person to see him coming and either say something or move out of the way. Dad also worried about coming up quickly behind a frail person; the cane would lightly touch them first, warning him of their presence so he could stop and avoid a collision. Residents often stopped suddenly in the middle of a hallway, and he was always on alert, fearful that he would knock someone down.

I swallowed hard when he requested help buying a cane. I'd never seen him use one, and it would be a tangible reminder that Admiral was gone. I agreed to call the Lighthouse for the Blind, where he received his diabetes education. I remembered seeing a small shop in the lobby where they sold aids for the blind, such as Braille clocks, measuring tapes, and playing cards. I'd check to ensure that they had a white cane in stock.

We went that afternoon to the Lighthouse. I watched Dad as he folded and unfolded the cane, explaining to the saleslady why he needed to buy one that day. Again, a large lump formed in my throat as he told her about Admiral. It felt surreal to be buying a cane; I still couldn't believe that he'd never walk with that beautiful dog again.

Dad and I walked slowly and in silence back up to his room. The hall felt empty and quiet without Admiral. I remembered the three of us together, how we'd taken up a lot of space in the halls or on a sidewalk, yet Admiral's cheerful presence was always reassuring and joyful.

Now it felt almost ghostly in his absence. I was sorry to say goodbye to Dad that night, knowing how empty the room would feel.

A few days later, Dad remarked to me about how much he missed Admiral. "It's hard because I keep seeing and feeling him, like he's still in the corner where he liked to lay. I developed a pattern of walking around him because he had certain places that he liked to lay, and I find myself still following that pattern. But I've had sixty-one good years of partnership with a dog, and I guess that I have no right to expect any more."

"Dad, maybe you could get another dog. Dr. Frei said that she'd write a supportive letter to the Seeing Eye. She believes that you could handle another dog. It's something to think about, and I'd help you if you needed it," I pleaded. I couldn't imagine him without a dog—I'd never known him without one.

"No, I'm too old for a young dog. He'd need lots of fast walks and exercise. I just couldn't keep up with him, and it wouldn't be fair to the dog. Besides, the training at the Seeing Eye is rigorous, and it would be too much for me. So, even though I know that you'd be willing to help, I'd still be responsible for all his care. No, it's better for me to use a cane," he said quietly, with a resigned tone.

"You know," he continued, "it's a little like going full circle. Shakespeare talked about the seven stages of man. Well, in a way that's me. I'm getting back into the field of mobility to where I was when I was fifteen. Of course, life was much simpler. Traffic moved slowly, there were no complex traffic signals or patterns, and there were a lot of people on the streets. If they saw me standing at a curb, they would lend me a hand if I needed it. Now I'm a lot older, it's too hard for me to go out alone, especially in Houston. I move too slowly, and the traffic won't stop for an old blind man. Besides, there's really no place that I can walk to—just a sidewalk that seems to go on forever."

"You know that I'll take you wherever you want or need to go."

"Thank you. Did I ever tell you what Jane used to say when she was failing?" Without waiting for an answer, he went on, "Well, you know how much she loved Admiral. She told me, 'When I get to heaven, I'm going to ask for a big gold Cadillac. I'll drive up there. Then I'll invite all the dogs we've had to go for a ride, because they all loved to ride. But Admiral will get the front seat beside me.' Who knows? If I get there and Admiral is sitting on the front seat beside her—I may just have to take him on my lap. I'd be glad to do that."

Unsure of what to say, I gave Dad a long hug and tried not to cry.

:• ••
   •

THANK YOU

ALTHOUGH HIS DIABETES was stable, the lymphoma that had been diagnosed five years earlier began to take its toll on his body. He never complained, but it must have frustrated and scared him to feel his body change and become weaker. At 92, he slept more during the day, often falling asleep in my living room easy chair.

"Oh! I must have drifted off a little. You know, your chair is just so comfortable."

"I know. That chair is dangerous. I often fall asleep in it while I'm trying to read. Mom always used to fall asleep there, and when she'd wake up, she said that she was just resting her eyes. I didn't believe that for a minute."

Dad required blood transfusions occasionally and injections to build up his white blood cells. He was hospitalized three times in six months for various complications. It seemed that almost every week we went to a doctor appointment at M.D. Anderson Cancer Center, and sometimes it took over half of a day from the time I picked him up until I left him safely in his room at Brighton Gardens.

Often, I'd bring him to my house for lunch after his appointments. He much preferred leftovers or a sandwich to the restaurant style meals in assisted living. He didn't complain about the food at

Brighton Gardens, but I know that he missed a home atmosphere. Living in a small studio and walking down to the dining room to eat at set times might have reminded him of being at the School for the Blind or Notre Dame. I wonder if he thought that his life had come full circle, that he was once again back in an institution. But now it was his permanent home, with only the end of his life to ponder, instead of being a young person with his life ahead of him.

I didn't mind the amount of time that I spent with Dad. I knew that he wouldn't live forever, and being with him was more important than my errands and chores. I wanted to be able to look back with a clear conscience that I had done all that I could to make his life and Mom's comfortable.

Although his body was frail, his mind was still very sharp. He insisted upon taking his own medications. Each bottle was labeled in Braille and kept in a special place in his closet. He knew when to take each medicine and refused all attempts by the Brighton Gardens nurses to help him. He was an unusual patient there; most residents couldn't keep track of their medicines and were dependent upon the nurses to bring their pills at the right time.

By the end of June 2006, it was apparent that the medications weren't doing enough. Dad was a great believer in "mind over matter," but his body began to fail, despite his best efforts. He became resigned to the idea of dying, and while his faith carried him through the spiritual aspects of the process, he was terrified that he'd suffer the worst possible death that he could conceive: drowning in his own secretions. He described nightmares where he couldn't breathe followed by waking up in a sweat. I could only try to reassure him that the doctor should be able to prevent that possibility, but I know that he remained unconvinced.

While waiting for Dr. Vu at his final doctor appointment, I fixed my gaze upon a close-up photo of a bright yellow sunflower. Evidently meant to provide cheer in an otherwise sterile exam room, it failed to lighten my mood. Dad and I sat on the hard plastic chairs. He was quiet, and I didn't feel like talking or attempting to entertain him as I had done during our many previous visits. Occasionally he breathed out a deep sigh and shifted position, but otherwise he seemed lost in his thoughts.

We heard a light tap and the door opened with a swoosh. Dad and I sat up straighter in our chairs and looked at her expectantly.

"Hello Mr. Pieroni! It's Dr. Vu. How are you doing?" she asked as she reached out to shake his pro-offered hand. She glanced at me and said "Hello," but clearly her eyes were on her patient. Doctor Vu sat down on the rolling stool and scooted almost knee-to-knee with him.

"Hello, doctor," he responded. "I'm doing about as well as could be expected, I guess."

"Do you have any pain?"

"No, no pain. Sometimes it's a little hard to breathe."

"Yes, well, you know that when you were in the hospital last week, we drained your right lung once and your left one twice. You had a lot of fluid, so that's why you had some trouble breathing."

"I know. Can you drain them again?"

"Unfortunately, no. The fluid would just come right back. Your body isn't able to excrete the fluid, even with the diuretics you've been taking. There's really nothing more that we can do."

Dad was silent for a moment. "Does that mean that I'll drown in my own secretions?" he asked with a shudder. "That just terrifies me."

"Oh no," Dr. Vu quickly tried to reassure him. "You'll get medicines from hospice that will keep you comfortable. We won't let you have a drowning sensation."

Dad didn't look convinced. "I don't understand how that will work, if you can't keep my lungs from filling up again."

"Well, you'll have oxygen if you need it, and the medicines will help with relaxing you. If you have any pain, they'll give you painkillers."

"Ok," he responded, still convinced that he would die while still struggling to breathe.

"Dad," I interrupted. "Remember that you have a caregiver staying with you twenty-four hours a day. She will help you with anything that you need and will call hospice if you need more medicine or whatever." Dad was a very private person and at first had resisted having someone else in the room. But he quickly realized the comfort of knowing that help was there if he needed her and seemed to enjoy the company and attention.

Dr. Vu reached for his hand and held it. I was touched that she was trying to reassure him, taking the time to be with a ninety-two-year-old man at his last doctor appointment. I swallowed hard, trying to keep from crying.

"You know," he said, "I've had a very good and long life. It wasn't easy, and sometimes it took every bit of energy I had to get through the day. But I don't have any regrets. I loved my wife and had her for over 58 years. I had a wonderful family. I wouldn't change a thing."

Dr. Vu smiled. "How did you meet your wife?"

Dad brightened and said, "Oh, well, we met at the Indiana School for the Blind back in the fourth grade. Would you like to hear the story?"

"Oh yes! Please tell it." Dr. Vu released his hand and sat up, waiting for him to begin.

Dad shifted in his chair, squared his shoulders, and began, "I was sitting at my desk—it was after Christmas, sometime in January—when the teacher said that a new girl would be joining the class. At that time, they were very strict about separating the boys from the girls. The boys were on one side of the classroom and the girls were on the other side. The next day, the new girl was seated right across the aisle from me. I couldn't talk to her, since there were strict rules about interacting with the opposite sex, but I loved it when she had to stand to recite, because then she stood right close to me in the aisle. I could have reached out and touched her, but of course that was forbidden.

"I still recall the first time that she made a big impression on me. She was asked to stand up and recite this poem:

So here hath been dawning
Another blue Day:
Think wilt thou let it
Slip useless away.
Out of Eternity
This new Day is born;
Into Eternity,
At night, will return."

When he finished, Doctor Vu looked wide-eyed at me, then back at Dad. "Oh my gosh! Do you remember that poem from hearing her say it once, back when you were in fourth grade?"

Smiling, he replied, "Oh yes. I've never forgotten that poem. I loved the sound of her voice."

"Who wrote it? Do you remember the title?"

"Thomas Carlyle is the author, and the title is *Today*."

"Wow." Dr. Vu looked at me in wonder. "How could you remember that for so many years? That's amazing. You must have an incredible memory."

"Maybe so, but it was when I first fell in love with Jane. Hearing her voice recite it over and over in my brain helped when we were apart, and I was lonely."

"That's so sweet. Well, Mr. Pieroni, it's been a pleasure having you as a patient. You have my cell phone number if you have any questions. Don't hesitate to call," she said as she stood to leave the room.

"Thanks for all you've done for me. You've been very helpful."

Dad and I slowly walked along corridors of M.D. Anderson Cancer Center, winding our way to the elevators. Although wheelchairs were plentiful in the clinic, Dad insisted on walking, saying, "I need the exercise." While I appreciated his desire to keep moving, his glacial pace tried my patience. We could have made it to the car so much quicker if he had agreed to the wheelchair. Now I understand that he was proud to walk on his own, and the extra fifteen minutes that it took was nothing compared to his feeling that even though he was dying, he still had the energy and desire to walk.

That night, I telephoned Frances Middleton at her home near Muncie. I told her that she needed to fly down quickly and that I'd arrange her flight. She agreed to come down the next day, which was Wednesday. Once plans were made, I called Dad to tell him the happy news of her impending arrival. He was delighted and surprised that I was able to get a flight for her so quickly.

"Have you talked to the people here? They usually have an extra room available for guests," he asked.

"Yes, it's all arranged. She'll be in room 287, just down the hall from you."

"Oh, that's wonderful. Thank you. I can't wait to see her."

At the airport, I anxiously awaited Frances' delayed flight. I was relieved when the elevator doors opened and saw Frances being pushed in a wheelchair. Although she was able to walk, she knew that it would be faster to have a ride to the Baggage Claim.

"Hello, Frances, it's good to see you. I am so glad that you could come so quickly," I said as I bent over to give her a hug.

"Oh, thank you for arranging everything. I can't wait to see Mario."

"And I know that he's very excited to see you, too."

It was almost seven o'clock when we arrived at Dad's room. He was dressed in his pajamas and bathrobe, sitting at his small table. The caregiver sat with him but excused herself to give them some privacy.

After exchanging greetings, Dad asked, "Are you hungry, Frances? I'm just making myself a peanut butter sandwich." He gestured to the toaster, where he was about to place two pieces of bread. A jar of peanut butter sat on the table, along with two glasses of water. "It's not very fancy, but I didn't feel like going downstairs for dinner," he explained.

"No, I'm not hungry, but I'm happy to sit with you," said Frances.

"Frances, how about if I show you your room and we can take your bag down there also," I asked. "Then you can come back and have an uninterrupted evening."

"That would be fine," she answered. "I'll be right back, Mario."

"Okay, I'll be right here."

After helping Frances to get settled, we walked back to Dad's room.

"Dad, I'm leaving now. I know that you have a lot to talk about," I said, smiling broadly.

"Okay. Good night, Mary."

"Good night, Dad. See you tomorrow, Frances."

"Thank you again, Mary. I really do appreciate all of your help," said Frances.

"I'm just happy that you got here! See you in the morning."

A few hours later, the ringing phone jolted me awake. I glanced at the clock: 4:42 a.m.

Nobody ever calls at that hour, and I knew that it was bad news. "Hello?"

"Miss Mary? This is Lila, your dad's caregiver. I'm afraid that Mr. Pieroni has passed away."

"What? When?"

"He died about 2:30. I've called hospice, and they'll be here soon."

I was in shock. The last time I'd seen him, he was eating a peanut butter sandwich and talking to Frances. How could he be dead? He was okay when I left him. And he was so happy to have Frances there.

"But what happened?" My mind couldn't grasp how he could have died so quickly.

"Well, he woke up about two o'clock and said that he had to go to the bathroom. So, I helped him walk to the bathroom, and then I got him back into bed. He said, 'thank you,' and I went back to sit on the couch. After a while I thought that he was being awfully quiet over there, so I went and checked on him. And he was gone."

"I'll be right there." I woke up Jeff and told him the news. "Do you want me to come with you?" he asked.

"No. I'll be okay. I need to go tell Frances."

Shortly after 5:00 a.m., I knocked on Frances' door. She opened it sooner than I expected and said, "Good morning!" with a big smile. She didn't seem to think that it was unusual for me to get her up that early.

I said, "It's not a good morning. Dad died a couple of hours ago."

"Oh no!" she exclaimed. "But he was fine last night. We talked about going down to breakfast this morning."

"I know. I can't believe it, either. Do you want to go see him?"

"Yes, let me put on my bathrobe."

We entered his room and paused. Already, his space felt different to me, as if the life spirit was drained. Frances and I walked to his bed and looked at his body lying motionless. I stared at his gray face, searching for any signs of life. Frances touched his arm, and I held his hand. It was cold. It was true. My father was gone. He didn't suffer. He didn't drown. I wondered if he could see what I looked like now, if he could finally see all that he had missed in his lifetime. I hoped that he and Mom were back together holding hands and going for a drive in her gold Cadillac with seven Seeing Eye dogs. Admiral would be in the front seat with Dad, joyously licking his hand. Together, they would drive off, delighted to be forever in each other's presence.

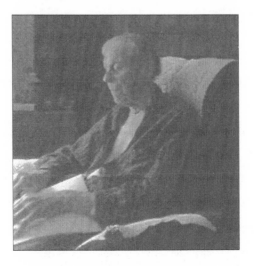

Reading Braille during his last hours

APPENDIX I

Following is the eulogy that I gave for my father at his funeral Mass July 17, 2006.

Good morning.

Thank you for coming to help celebrate my father's life. I am Mary Harper, the baby of the family. I've known my Dad for almost 53 years, but it wasn't until 8 years ago that I had the privilege of really getting to know him. It was 1998 when my parents decided to give up their beautiful Chapel Hill, North Carolina home and move to Houston. My mother was not well, and maintaining their home was becoming too difficult. I watched my Dad as he lovingly helped my Mom through the last year of her life. He was always so kind and loving toward the woman he first met as the new girl in fourth grade at the Indiana School for the Blind. Not long ago, he told his doctor about the day that Jane recited a poem in school. He then recited the same poem as if it were yesterday. I wish that I'd written the poem down, but at the time I didn't have any paper, and my memory isn't nearly as good as my Dad's.

Dad had a phenomenal memory. He memorized not only poems, but music. Dad played the piano and violin by memorizing each measure of music. He memorized thick law books at the University of Notre Dame and then took the state bar exam orally. I can't imagine sitting there, facing those examiners and having to answer many complex legal questions. Dad passed with flying colors.

For being totally blind, he had an amazing sense of direction. He memorized all the streets in Muncie, knew the county road system and almost all of the state highways. He knew all the counties and county seats in the state of Indiana and could tell you the best way to get to a particular place. Years ago, a local newspaper columnist wrote about the time an acquaintance was driving my Dad downtown. Apparently, the man was distracted talking to Dad, and he began driving the wrong way on a one-way street. Dad said "Hey! Aren't you going the wrong way?" The man was amazed, and I believe a bit embarrassed, that a blind man saved him from a possible accident.

When Dad moved to Chapel Hill, he quickly learned his way around the town. He walked with his dogs Job and then Admiral all through the neighborhood for exercise and to run errands. In Houston, even though he no longer took long neighborhood walks, he still wanted to learn as much as possible about the city and its layout. As we drove around Houston, he'd ask where we were and where the street went and quickly learned the major streets.

Dad also memorized voices. Growing up, I was amazed at how many people would say, "Hello, Mario!" and he'd say, "Hello, George! How are you?" He always got the name right.

I learned so much from my Dad.

I developed patience, particularly in the last few years of his life, as he moved slower and slower.

I got my sense of humor from him. He could usually see the funny side of life.

He taught me to be kind to all, no matter the race or economic status of the person. He spent hours helping me to learn how to write class papers. I give him credit for the

A's I received on those papers in philosophy class.

Dad taught me to not put off living, to enjoy what you have today, and to not be afraid to reach for what you want.

He was a great example of how regularly exercising can keep you healthy. Many of you may remember him walking home from work, which gave himself and one of his seven Seeing Eye dogs some great exercise. I think that it was also a way for him to let go of the stresses of the day so that he could relax at home and be present for his family. One of my fondest childhood memories is of just the two of us going for a walk on a cold winter's night, crunching through the snow. When I complained about the cold, he said that it was "invigorating," and to breathe deeply. My dad never missed an opportunity to teach me a new word.

But perhaps most of all, he taught me to love. My father had a great capacity for love. He loved and cared my mother for fifty-seven years. Dad worked hard as an attorney and judge, while Mom worked hard to raise four children. On the face of it, there's nothing remarkable about that. But considering that they led such normal lives while completely blind, well, I think that's pretty amazing.

Dad made all of his own financial decisions but needed my help to pay the bills and balance the checkbook. A few years after my mother passed, I began to notice more and more long-distance phone calls to a certain number in Muncie. Then Dad decided to travel more frequently to Muncie, ostensibly to visit my sister Anne. He would fly up by himself, and Anne and Sue picked him up at the airport. Every trip to Muncie included a visit with his former secretary and court reporter, Frances Middleton. Their friendship grew and once again, my dad showed how much love he had within. Frances brought him much joy and helped him through the last difficult months of his illness.

He loved to travel, and after my mom passed, we took many trips together. We went to Wisconsin to visit my sister Rita, stayed in a cabin in the mountains of Colorado, enjoyed the Pacific Ocean in southern California, made snowballs in the mountains of Utah, picked up shells on Sanibel Island, Florida, and even spent a week in the rainforest of Belize. He loved the birds that sang outside our cabin and enjoyed a day exploring the Mayan ruins. I'm so glad that we took those trips. I have so many wonderful memories, and I know that he truly enjoyed anticipating them and then remembering the experiences afterwards.

My Dad loved dogs, books, listening to and making tapes for friends, chocolate, fried catfish, going for rides in cars, trains, and boats, telling stories, and National Public Radio. He loved music, and I took him to many Houston Symphony concerts. I liked to watch his hands as he listened to the concert. He would often look as if he were directing, using subtle hand movements, but he was fully involved with the music.

I'll miss my dad, but I have many wonderful memories to sustain me. I'm so grateful for his love, and the example that he set will continue to influence me and, I hope, everyone else who knew him.

I will close by quoting from the book of Micah:

This is what
The Lord asks of you, Only this;
To act justly
To love tenderly,
And walk humbly With your God.

APPENDIX II

Charles' Eulogy

I have always been proud of my brother. My parents came here from Italy, and I was born a year later and three years before Mario.

You can imagine my parents' concern when they learned Mario was blind, as at that time, blind people couldn't earn a living. Most citizens thought a blind person was one standing on the corner selling pencils.

I grew up with Mario as my best friend, and we did everything together. [All brothers aren't that close.] As a result, I grew up not really realizing that Mario was handicapped. For instance, I bought my first car when I was 15, and the first thing I did was teach Mario how to drive. It was a convertible, and Mario would sit in the driver's seat, and I would sit in the rumble seat and put my hands on his shoulders in order to give him directions. This allowed me to direct him which way to turn by applying pressure on one side or the other. To stop, Id' press both shoulders. We could also use oral instructions. Drivers licenses weren't required at the time, and on Sundays, we'd take our friends on rides to the country.

Mario was 12, then, and driving! People around town knew what we were doing, so they watched out for us!

We took many trips together. When I was 18 and Mario 15, we went to Italy for 10 months, where the two of us traveled by train all over the country.

Mario developed a great self-confidence, and with both of us, he could do about anything.

One of my great pleasures was to see Mario graduate from Notre Dame law school, where he was the first blind student to accomplish this feat. After graduation, he started business as a junior partner in my practice, where he did most of the trial work and I did most of the office work. We made such a good team that our business grew to the point where we took on four more Notre Dame law school graduates.

Our years together were, in fact, an expression of our family relationships. Our practice was successful, and my parents were able to witness Mario prosper on his own and become a successful attorney, judge, and family man.

It has been a ninety-two-year privilege living, working, and relating with my brother Mario. He has been a lifelong friend, and always an inspiration. He taught me the virtue of perseverance. He embodied the teaching of acceptance of things you can't change and the courage to change those that you can. Mario knew the difference.

Time takes a toll on all of us, and due to my diminished physical condition, I am unable to attend his internment, but in spirit, we are, as always, united.

APPENDIX III

Tribute to Mario Pieroni
September 25, 1970

The Indiana Easter Seal Society also wishes to pay tribute to you, Mario, and to thank you for the many years of service you have given the Societies for Crippled Children and Adults-the years you served on the State Board and then as President and now as legal advisor,—for traveling over the state in the early days of the State Society helping to organize local societies and for the faithful service you have given your Delaware County Society.

It is said, "Many men owe the grandeur of their lives to their tremendous difficulties." You have truly experienced difficulties, and your life has sown majesty and graciousness. Ralph Waldo Emerson observed, "When it is dark enough men see the stars." Mario, you have known the darkness and seen the whole Milky Way.

You have always looked on the positive side of life—seeing what you do for others rather than what they could do for you.

Robert Schuller's words aptly describe your philosophy, "Look not at what you have lost but what you have left." "Look"—How many times we have heard you say, "Oh, I'm so glad to see you," and we knew you were truly seeing, —perhaps, more than others would ever see in us. We have heard you tell of going to Notre Dame to "see" the football games. We'll never forget your telling of "The beautiful flight to Boston for a National Convention."

Mario, we stand humble before your achievements. You have been an inspiration to all whose paths you have crossed. We thank you and may God continue to Bless You and Yours.

Mary Alice Eisaman (Mrs. Jack L.)

APPENDIX IV

Frances Middleton's Remembrances

In October 1964 Pieroni, Hynes, Dixon & Marsh contacted VanLandingham Employment Agency and told them of their need for a secretary. They sent me for an interview with Mario Pieroni. We had a rather short interview, and Mario asked me to work for a short time as a trail period to see how we worked together. That lasted for more than 14 years, first at the law office and then 8 years at the courthouse.

Mario was a very kind and considerate person. He realized that I had not done office work for some 20 or more years and was very patient while I adjusted to the routine. Fortunately, my typing and shorthand came back very quickly. (He let me know immediately that he did not want to dictate to a machine.) We read back all the documents and letters that he dictated—it helped him to review the material and make sure everything was just right, and it also helped me to catch any errors I might have made. He had a rubber stamp he used to sign any papers. He followed that same practice as Judge. The attorneys usually prepared their own Orders for the Judge's signature, and Mario was careful to have them read to him before he signed them. One time at the courthouse an out-of-town attorney objected to the use of the stamp on an Order. He said that would not be acceptable. He refused to accept my explanations, so I introduced him to the Judge. I don't know what was said, but there were no further problems.

We spent many hours in the law libraries, both at the office and at the courthouse. He seemed to know just which books we needed to look at and was always willing to explain to me some of the issues involved. The search was always an enjoyable time.

Mario was the attorney for the Delaware County Department of Public Welfare, and it was part of the job to handle the estates when a recipient died. In order to qualify for welfare, a recipient was required to relinquish ownership of any real estate to the Department, and then when the recipient died, the property was sold and the proceeds went to the Department. One time we received a deed for such a property that was being sold, and Mario was to approve it on behalf of the Department. We read the document, including the real estate description. Mario would follow the description by putting his finger on one place on his desk (as the starting point) and then move a finger on the other hand according to the direction and length given in the description. We read the description once, and something seemed not quite right, so we went through it again. Sure enough, he did not end up at the starting point. I don't know how many attorneys and possibly abstractors had seen that description, but it took a blind attorney to find the mistake.

Other than reading there were very few things Mario couldn't do for himself. Sometimes when he returned from lunch he would ask me to check to make sure he had not spilled something on his clothes. Also, I found that I could not say his dog's name in the dog's presence. Sometimes I drove him home from work, but sometimes he preferred to walk. At those times, we left the office together, but when we went our separate ways, we never said goodbye. He just quietly went on with his dog, and I turned the other way.

At the time Mario was Judge, Superior Court No. 1 had only civil jurisdiction—no criminal matters, probate, or juvenile. Many of the cases were divorce. Friday was known as "hate day" in all three of the courts having that jurisdiction in the county.

Except for the reading Mario did not need much additional help, but it was different working for Mario. He seemed more considerate than most people, and always had the right words to say. In the courtroom, he showed compassion and was always courteous. He had a way of making a person feel that their ideas and thoughts were important.

He was a person of high ideals and convictions and was not afraid to live up to them. The world would be a much better place if we had more people like him.

Every time I talked with Mario, I felt that I was a better person just for knowing him.

Frances Middleton

APPENDIX V

Blizzard of '78

Note: My father was an excellent storyteller. He recorded this story on his cassette tape recorder, ,and after transcribing it, I realized that it should be told in his own words. The following is lightly edited.

Mario: I've always had a good sense of direction. It was critical for me, since I often walked alone or with my dog. My dog wouldn't know where I wanted to go. I had to tell him. Some people think that guide dogs just know where to take their master. That's not true. The master is in charge and tells the dog which way to turn. The dog takes the master around objects that are in the way and stops at curbs. He can't tell if the light is green. I have to listen to determine if it's safe to cross.

Sometimes I'd walk to work. Leaving the house, I turned left onto the sidewalk and walked down the north side of Jackson Street. I crossed a number of side streets. Of course, I knew the names of every street. After about fifteen minutes, I arrived at the bridge over White River and kept right on going. Eventually, I'd come right down into the center of town, to Walnut Street. It was the main north–south street in downtown. That's where I turned left and went two blocks north. My office was on the northeast corner of Washington and Walnut. When I left the firm, I went to the courthouse diagonally across the street, so it was about a block closer to home.

I actually walked home more than I walked to the office since the morning had more time constraints. Usually, I'd leave the house about eight o'clock, turn left, and go up to the first street east. There was a light there, so I could cross with the traffic. I'd go and stand on the opposite corner, and the bus would come from the west, stop, and pick me up. Sometimes an acquaintance would stop and roll down their window and say, "Hey Mario! Do you want a ride?" I'd often accept their offer, especially if it was cold or raining.

When I ride with someone, I have a keen awareness of where we are. If I fall into a conversation and become absent-minded, then I can get lost, and I just can't let that happen. One day, I was riding with a fellow and I realized that he was going the wrong way down a one-way street. That's an awful feeling! I didn't want to embarrass him, but I also didn't want to get into an accident. So I asked him, "Aren't we on a one-way street, going the wrong way?" He quickly realized his mistake and turned down a side street. The poor guy felt kind of sheepish, but he must have told a newspaper friend about it. The story got published in the local paper and then picked up by the Associated Press. I got letters and clippings from all over the Midwest and even Florida. I was amazed that people liked that story.

I'm terrified of becoming lost. I have nightmares where I've become absent-minded on a walk with my dog and I've forgotten to take notice of the cues that tell me where I am. I'm wandering around mad at myself and listening for something familiar. I can't figure out where I am and panic. That's when I wake up sweating, my heart pounding.

The last winter we lived in Muncie, there was one especially bad blizzard when everything was shut down. I was home for several days, and it was bitterly cold with heavy snow. Well, I wasn't interested in going out. There was practically no traffic on Jackson Street except just people that had to be out. I had to, of course, take my dog out.

I'd always taken him down to a vacant field, which was—well, I'd leave the house and take the back alley down to the corner of Cole Street. Then go up Cole Street half a block and there across the street was a large vacant area—it was a perfect place to take the dog. So we always went there.

When the snow got too deep, I had to take him out in the back yard because nothing was cleared. But the time came when some cars had made it through the alley. I thought, *Well, it's so still and quiet out tonight, I think that we'll just go back there to the field. Take a little walk.* We were both underworked and needed some exercise.

We found the car tracks and followed them down to the corner. Of course, I knew where the street was by listening to the acoustics bouncing off of the garages. (I often made clicking noises to determine how close an object was—similar to how a bat uses echolocation.) We turned north on Cole, found some tracks, and sort of soldiered along. Finally, we got to the field. I put the dog on a long leash and let him sort of run around until he got finished. It was time to start back, but I had absent-mindedly been following him. I was turned around, and suddenly, I didn't know which way was which.

I was out in the open. At times like that, I rely on certain sounds. There's a busy street a couple of blocks to the west, and Jackson Street is one block south. In normal circumstances, I could hear the traffic and orient myself. In the daytime, I can feel the sun or know which way the wind is blowing. But there was nothing this time. No wind, no sun, no traffic. Just absolute stillness and very cold!

I put on his harness and said, "Let's go home." But he wasn't interested in going home. He was so underworked that he wanted to run. He wanted to go anywhere. I said, "Okay, we'll start, and I'll get a cue." We walked down some tracks, but I got no cues. For one thing, snow mutes everything. I couldn't bounce any sound off of buildings. I didn't know where to find the street. Curbs normally help me to know my exact location, but they were covered with snow.

Even my dog, who is trained to stop at curbs, couldn't find them. We continued trudging through the drifts; I listened carefully and hopefully for a familiar sound.

We went a distance. I didn't know which way we were going, but I knew where each of the four directions would ultimately take us. If we went the right way, I would come out to Jackson Street. I should get a cue there to know which way to turn. Or if I went north, eventually we'd get into the hospital. But that was quite a distance away, and it would be very confusing. I figured that we had to keep moving; my dog was happy to oblige.

I was starting to get really cold and worried. There were some houses in the area, but they would be hard to find in the snow. That's the last thing that I would want to subject my pride to. I'd have to try to find somebody and knock on a door or a window—whatever I could find—and hope that there'd be somebody home that would respond. I'd have to say, "Gee, I'm lost." That's just something that would be intolerable.

I walked quite some distance it seemed, and I still couldn't figure out where I was.

Desperation was setting in. So, I said, "Let's turn around and try a different way." I'm not sure just which way we went, but I think that we went west on a little street. We came to a place where the car tracks sort of crossed, and I think that I was beginning to get a subconscious notion of where I was because I said, "Let's turn left."

We went a little way, and I began to hear the sound of a motor. A block west from our house, there was a grocery on the corner.

They used to leave some kind of a fan running in back of the store; I recognized the sound and then I knew exactly where I was. Few times in my life have I been more relieved.

We walked around in front of the store. I was glad that the walk was partly cleared off.

There was no question that I'd get home. But on the way, I got to thinking: I could have wandered around back there, and no one would have seen me. Eventually, I might have fallen in the snow or become weakened with the cold. Jane would be at home, not suspecting that anything unusual was going on. I went out every night. Some nights I walked and other nights I'd stop over next door at my parents. She wouldn't likely sound the alarm for some time. I thought, *Wouldn't it be awful to perish within a block of your house?* I never told Jane about my harrowing walk. I've never told anybody until now. I didn't want it to get into the newspaper. I could see the headline: *Judge Pieroni Gets Lost in Snow*. My pride had suffered enough.

APPENDIX VI

APPLICATION.

To the Superintendent of the Indiana Institution for the Education of the Blind:

The undersigned, desiring to procure the admission of a pupil for education in the Institution under your charge, would submit for your consideration the following particulars in answer to the several interrogatories herein propounded, and will stand pledged for the correctness of the same, as well as for the proper fulfillment of the requirements set forth in the circular prefixed hereto:

1. *What is the REAL and full name of the applicant?* Ans. **Mario Pieroni**

2. *In what State or County was applicant born?* Ans. **Muncie, Indiana.**

3. *What is the date of the applicant's birth?* Ans. **January 24, 1914.**

4. *At what age did the blindness occur?* Ans. **Soon after birth**

5. *What is the supposed cause of blindness?* Ans. **Infantile Glaucoma.**

6. *Is the blindness total?* Ans. **Yes.**

7. *If it is not total, is it sufficient to prevent the acquirement of an education in a school for the seeing?* Ans. **Yes**

8. *Is the applicant of sound mind and susceptible to intellectual culture.* Ans. **Yes**

9. *Has the applicant any bodily deformity or infirmity, and if so, what?* Ans. **None.**

10. *What is the applicant's general state of health?* Ans. **Good.**

11. *Has applicant epilepsy or any infectious disease?* Ans. **No**

12. *Has the applicant ever been a pupil in any other school for the blind, and if so, what one and how long?* Ans. **No.**

13. *Is applicant free from all immoral habits?* Ans. **Yes**

14. *What are the full names of the OWN parents of the applicant?* Ans.
    Antonio Pieroni – Eletta Pieroni.

15. *Were such parents related before marriage, and if so, how?* Ans. **No**

16. *Are there other cases of blindness in the family, and if so, how are they related to the applicant? Ans.* No

17. *If the father of the applicant is not living, or has, for any reason, ceased to provide for the same, who is his or her present guardian? Ans.* --

18. *What is the postoffice address of the father or guardian, as the case may be, of the applicant? Ans.* 400 E. Charles St., Muncie, Indiana.

19. *What are the names of the Township, County and State in which the applicant has legal residence? Ans.* Center Township- Delaware County- Indiana.

20. *If in the State of Indiana, what is the name of the present Trustee of such Township? Ans.* Merritt Heath

21. *Make any special statement regarding applicant that is needful for a full understanding of the case.*

22. *White or colored? Ans.* White

Signed this 28th *day of* August *A. D.* 1922.

Antonio Pieroni
(To be signed on above line)

The State of Indiana, Delaware County, ss:

I, the undersigned, Justice of the Peace in and for said County, hereby certify that Mario Pieroni *the above named applicant for admission as a pupil of the Indiana Institution for the Education of the Blind, is a legal resident of the Township and County herein set forth as the residence of said applicant.*

WITNESS my hand, this 28 *day of* Augst *, A.D.* 1922

Edward W. Swain

JUSTICE OF THE PEACE

APPLICATION

To the Board of Trustees of the Indiana School for the Blind:

The undersigned, desiring to procure the admission of a child for education in the School under your charge, submits for your consideration answers to the following questions, and will be responsible for the fulfillment of the requirements set forth in the circular prefixed hereto:

1. What is the full name of the child for whom admission into this School is desired? Ans. *Ella Jane Ingall*

2. In what State and County was it born? Ans. *Indiana, Wabash Co.*

3. What is the date of its birth? Ans. *Sept. 9, 1913.*

4. At what age did the blindness occur? Ans. *Birth*

5. What is the cause of blindness? Ans. *Unknown*

6. Is the blindness total? Ans. *No.*

7. If it is not total, is it sufficient to prevent the acquirement of an education in a school for the seeing? Ans. *Yes*

8. Is the child of sound mind, and susceptible of intellectual culture? Ans. *Yes*

9. Has it any bodily deformity or infirmity, and if so, what? Ans. *No*

10. What is its general state of health? Ans. *Good*

11. Has it epilepsy or any infectious or contagious disease? Ans. *No*

12. Has it been a pupil in any school for the blind, and if so, what one and how long? Ans. *No*

13. Has it been a pupil in any school for the seeing, and if so, how long? Ans. *Yes Five years*

14. Is the child free from all immoral habits? Ans. *Yes*

15. What are the full names of the parents of the child? Ans. *Charlie Clayton Ingall & Bessie Edith Ingall*

16. Were such parents related before marriage, and if so, how? Ans. *No*

17. Are there other cases of blindness in the family, and if so, how are they related to the child? Ans. *No*

18. If the parents of the child are not living, or have ceased to provide for same, who is its present guardian?

Ans.

19. What is the postoffice address of the parents or guardian, as the case may be, of the child? Ans.

Wabash, Ind.   RR # 8

20. What are the names of the Township and County in which the child has legal residence? Ans.

Noble Township, Wabash County

21. What is the name of the present Trustee of such Township? Ans. *W. G. Gardner*

22. Is the child white or colored? Ans. *White*

23. What helpful information, not covered by the above answers, can you give regarding the child? Ans.

THE STATE OF INDIANA, *Wabash* COUNTY, SS:

I hereby solemnly swear, or affirm, that the answers given above are true to the best of my information and belief, and that I will fulfill all requirements stated in this application.

(Individual Name) *Charlie C. Small*

Subscribed and sworn to before me, this *15* day of *September* 192*4*

Ellis Bloomer,

Justice of the Peace

(Official Title.)

THE STATE OF INDIANA, *Wabash* COUNTY, SS:

I, the undersigned, Justice of the Peace in and for said County, hereby certify that

Ella Jane Long

(Name of Child)

the above described child, is a legal resident of the Township and County set forth above as the residence of said child.

WITNESS my hand and seal, this *15* day of *September* 192*4*

Ellis Bloomer

(Justice of the Peace.)

INDIANA SCHOOL FOR THE BLIND

INDIANAPOLIS, INDIANA

INFORMATION

1. The purpose of this School is purely educational, and it is in no sense an asylum or a home. The aim is to give a practical education to the young blind of both sexes residing in the State. The common and the high school branches are taught, and thorough instruction is given in industrial trades such as broom-making, cane-seating chairs, piano tuning, etc. The girls learn sewing by hand and machine, knitting, crocheting, beadwork, etc. The intention is to make the pupils useful, contented, and self-supporting citizens. An extensive course in music is available to all that have talent in this direction. Instruction is given on the piano, organ, violin, mandolin, etc. A thorough course is given in vocal training. A gymnasium is equipped, and a special teacher drills the pupils in systematic physical exercises. Pupils when not under control of teachers are in charge of governesses.

2. The school year commences on the fourth Wednesday of September, and continues in session thirty-six weeks.

3. Persons under eight or over twenty-one years of age are not admitted.

4. No person of imbecile or unsound mind or of confirmed immoral character will be knowingly received into the School; and in case any pupil shall, after a fair trial, prove incompetent for instruction or disobedient to the regulations of the School, such pupil will be thereupon discharged.

5. The School is maintained by the State: and tuition, board, and washing are furnished free of cost to all pupils. The parents or friends of pupils or proper officials must supply them with suitable clothing in such quantity as will admit of necessary changes. Each article of clothing should be distinctly marked with the owner's name, and must be sent in good condition. The traveling expenses of the pupils must be defrayed by parents, friends, or proper officials.

6. It is positively required that every pupil shall be removed from the School at the close of the school year and at such other times as may be deemed necessary by the proper officers of the School.

7. Persons bringing pupils to the School or visiting them while here can not be accommodated with board and lodging by the School.

8. All letters to the pupils should be addressed in care of the School in order to insure their prompt delivery.

9. Anyone desiring the admission of a child must fill the subjoined form of application, and forward the same to the Superintendent of the School, giving truthful answers to the interrogatories therein contained. The appended affidavit and certificate must be properly filled; and the child must, in no case, be sent until notice has been received by the applicant that such child is eligible.

10. The Superintendent will cheerfully give information in regard to the School, and will thankfully receive any information concerning those that should be receiving its benefits.

GEO. S. WILSON,
Superintendent.

SUGGESTIONS

To the Parents and the Guardians of Blind Children.

1. Eligible blind children, unless under the most favorable circumstances at home, should be in this School at eight years of age.

2. Teach them to take plenty of exercise in the open air, to go errands, and to be as active and helpful as possible.

3. Do not permit the blindness of children to make you less strict in securing obedience, cleanliness, and politeness. Especially should their physical growth be so guarded that they may possess healthy, symmetrical bodies, and may be free from any peculiarity of movement, such as the nervous twitching of arms and fingers, and turning of heads.

4. Permit the blind children to enjoy all the privileges granted other children. Let blind children attend the public school, the Sunday school, the church services, places of amusement, etc.

5. Teach them the names, forms, and uses of common objects around them.

6. An embossed alphabet and an embossed primer will be furnished on request, from which the blind children may be taught the letters and simple words. Blind children may attend the public schools a year or two with advantage, and, with little inconvenience to the teacher, may do well the same work as seeing classmates.

7. When pupils enter the school, health permitting, they should attend punctually and regularly until the course is completed.

8. Forbid blind children the use of tobacco, intoxicants, etc.

9. Do not dwell upon the misfortune of blind children in their presence, nor permit others to do so. Encourage blind children to be cheerful, hopeful, and industrious.

10. It has been demonstrated that the majority of blind men and women, if intelligent and deserving, can make a living and do a creditable part in any community. Instead of being helpless burdens, they become self-supporting and self-respecting, a source of gratification rather than of care and regret to their friends.

(Do not write in the space below.)

Accepted, _9/19/1924_ .... Rejected.

Date of Entrance, ... _Term 1924-5_ ....
(DATE)

Date of Permanent Withdrawal, ...

Remarks: _1st or original application on which 1st admission was based_

ACKNOWLEDGEMENTS

THIS BOOK TOOK over ten years to write. It began in a memoir writing class as a long chapter filled with facts about my parents and growing up in a home where our parents couldn't see us. Thanks to the help of those initial class members, especially Louise Deretchin and Maria Zerr, the manuscript slowly expanded.

The book went through several drafts, which were helpfully critiqued by members of my writing group: Aline Myers, Betty Jo Hall, and Louise Deretchin. This book is improved immeasurably by their thoughtful comments, questions, and suggestions.

My late sister, Anne Szopa, read many early chapters and contributed her memories to the stories. We spent hours emailing or talking on the phone, comparing our perspectives as she was the first-born and ten years older than me. We realized that we actually grew up in very different families. She had different responsibilities and had more expectations placed on her than I did as the youngest. I cherish the times that we had together and wish that she was alive to see this publication.

My sister, Rita DeBoth, also provided immeasurable help by clarifying some of my memories and adding her thoughts. Since Rita is only three years older than me, we shared many of the same experiences. This book provided an opportunity for us to share memorable moments of our childhood.

Thanks to my brother, John Pieroni, for his encouraging emails and contributing his memories. This book would not be complete without them.

Extended family also were extremely helpful. My cousin, Lisa Vergara, thoughtfully critiqued an earlier draft. Her insights contributed significantly to the next draft. Another cousin, Kevin Ganster, provided photos, letters, and encouragement. He also critiqued an early draft, correcting errors and giving ideas for the next version. Kevin is a treasure-trove of Pieroni history, and I thank him for his generous sharing.

A special thanks to my nephew, Vincent Szopa, who critiqued numerous drafts and always inspired me to continue. His technical help with formatting saved my sanity several times.

Although not technically a member of the Pieroni family, I'd like to thank the late Frances Middleton for her memories of working with my father. Her words appear in Appendix IV and give another view of my father that only someone who worked closely with him could write.

This book would not have been possible without the insights of two editors that helped tame the words swirling around my brain. Leslie Contreras Schwartz and Cynthia Johnson both contributed their time and expertise to helping me organize my writing. Their comments and questions helped to shape the book and I'm most grateful.

I am indebted to the kind staff of the Indiana School for the Blind, who gave me a tour of their beautiful campus. It was thrilling for me to walk the same halls that my parents had walked ninety years before, and to see the beautiful theater where they had held their clandestine meetings during rehearsals. All records of my parents' era are now stored at the Indiana State Archives. I was surprised and delighted that they found both of my parents' applications from 1922 and 1924!

My late husband, Jeff Harper, was an early champion of this book. His critiques of the first drafts encouraged me to keep going. He cooked every dinner, enabling me to take that time to write. I miss his cooking, his smile, and his love.

I am so fortunate to have a partner who loves to read and doesn't mind reading my later drafts. His suggestions have improved my writing and I'm so grateful for his time and expertise. Thomas Heffner, who also likes to cook, has fed me both physically and spiritually. Thanks for always being there for me.

ABOUT THE AUTHOR

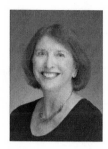 MARY HARPER IS a retired social worker and author of *The Sound of Her Voice: My Blind Parents' Story*. A native of Muncie, Indiana, she is a graduate of the University of Virginia and earned her Master's in Social Work from the University of Houston.

She lives in Houston, TX with her two rescue cats. Myrrh had been dumped in a rural area and was found on Christmas Day, 2008. Lily was adopted shortly after the kitten's infected eyes were removed; the fearless kitty has no problem jumping onto furniture or Mary's lap. Her cats were comforting when Mary's husband, Jeff, passed away in 2012.

Mary has two adult children and loves being a grandmother.

To contact Mary, send an email to mary@marypharper.com.

Follow Mary on social media:

Facebook: @MaryHarperAuthor
Instagram: @mary_p_harper